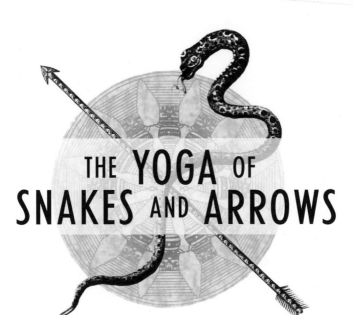

THE YOGA OF
SNAKES AND ARROWS

Other Books by Harish Johari

Attunements for Dawn and Dusk (Audio)

Attunements for Day and Night (Audio)

Ayurvedic Healing Cuisine

Ayurvedic Massage

Breath, Mind, and Consciousness

Chakras

Dhanwantari

The Healing Power of Gemstones

Numerology

The Planet Meditation Kit

Sounds of Tantra (Audio)

Sounds of The Chakras (Audio)

Tools for Tantra

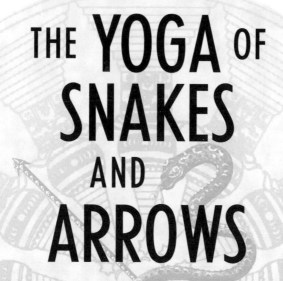

THE YOGA OF SNAKES AND ARROWS

THE LEELA OF SELF-KNOWLEDGE

Harish Johari

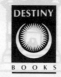

Destiny Books
Rochester, Vermont

Destiny Books
One Park Street
Rochester, Vermont 05767
www.DestinyBooks.com

Destiny Books is a division of Inner Traditions International

Originally published in 1975 by Coward, McCann & Geoghegan under the title *Leela: The Game of Self-Knowledge*
Second edition published in 1993 as a boxed set with game board by Destiny Books
Third edition published in 2007 by Destiny Books under the title *The Yoga of Snakes and Arrows*

Library of Congress Cataloging-in-Publication Data

Johari, Harish, 1934–1999.
    The yoga of snakes and arrows : the leela of self-knowledge / Harish Johari.
        p. cm.
    Originally published: New York : Coward, McCann & Geoghegan, 1975.
    ISBN-13: 978-1-59477-178-1 (pbk.)
    ISBN-10: 1-59477-178-2 (pbk.)
    1. Leela (Game) 2. Games—Religious aspects—Hinduism. 3. Hinduism—Doctrines. I. Title.
    GV1469.L44J639 2007
    793.93—dc22

                                                                2007014065

ISBN of current title *The Yoga of Snakes and Arrows:* ISBN-13: 978-1-59477-178-1

ISBN-10: 1-59477-178-2

Printed and bound in China by Reliance Printing Co., Ltd.

10   9   8   7   6

Text design by Virginia L. Scott Bowman
This book was typeset using Sabon with Agenda and Agenda Condensed as the display typefaces

Contents

The Commentaries

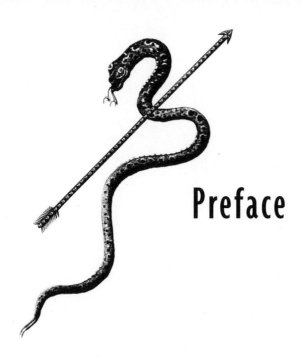

Preface

The Yoga of Snakes and Arrows is based on Leela, a game in which each of us is a player acting out his role. Leela is the universal play of cosmic energy. It is divine play that is present in the nature of the Supreme Self. It is this playful nature that creates the world of names and forms—the phenomenal world. Leela is life itself, energy expressed as the myriad forms and feelings presented continuously to the self.

The essence of the player is his ability to become, to adopt a role. That which is the essence of the player can enter into any role. But once the player enters into the game, once he assumes the identity of the persona he adopts, he loses sight of his true nature. He forgets the essence of what it is to play the game. His moves are decided by the karma die.

As there are moments when sunlight momentarily illumines the patterns of waves, and flows in a river, so too there are moments when the clear light of consciousness reveals the patterns in the player's life role. At those moments the nature and flow of life energy stands forth as though in relief. At those moments the player loses his attachment to his role and begins to see his life as a part of a larger whole.

The purpose of Leela is to help the player gain this ability to withdraw from his identifications and see how he might become a better player. For the game of Leela is a microcosm of the larger game of self-knowledge. Contained within the seventy-two spaces of the game board is the essence of thousands of years of self-exploration, the heart of Indian tradition.

As the player moves from space to space, square to square, he begins to see patterns in his own existence, emerging with ever-deepening clarity as his understanding of the game broadens. His sense of detachment grows as he sees each state as temporary, something to move beyond. And once the temporality of any space becomes a reality for the player, he can detach from that space and let it go as he seeks to discover ever more about the wonder that is Being.

As with all games, here too there is a goal, an object to be attained. Because the essence of the player is his ability to identify, his only chance of "winning" the game is to identify with that which is his Source. This is Cosmic Consciousness, the essence of pure Being, which transcends time and space, knows no limits, and is infinite, absolute, eternal, changeless, the All, without attributes, beyond both name and form. The game ends when the player becomes himself, the essence of play.

The saints who invented the game of Leela used the game board to recognize the present state of their own being. By observing their course of movement from one plane to another they could practically observe which snakes brought them down and which arrows took them up. The moves were decided by a karmic die, yet the die when thrown indicated their own evolution because it represented the present state of the player. They consciously observed the pattern through which they were moving, by playing the game time and again and watching carefully their own reaction while landing on a snake or an arrow. Observing their own inner self, they could tell whether they had understood what it is to be not involved. At the same time, the network of the game gave them a deeper insight into the principle of the divine knowledge on which the game board was based. It was a study of scriptures and discovery of the self at the same time. This is the uniqueness of Leela, the yoga of snakes and arrows, the game of self-knowledge.

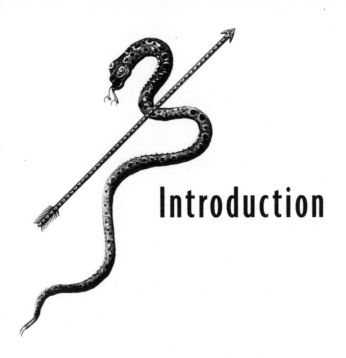

Introduction

Originally called Gyan Chaupad (literally *Gyan* = knowledge; *Chaupad* = a game played with dice: so "Game of Knowledge"), the game Leela was designed by the seers and saints as a key to inner states and to learn the principles of *dharma*[1]*—usually called Hinduism. With its snakes and arrows and seventy-two squares representing seventy-two planes, the game provides a key to the knowledge of the Vedas,[2] the Shrutis,[3] the Smiritis,[4] and the Puranas.[5] Playing the game is playing with the manifested divine knowledge found in the aphorisms and doctrines of yoga,[6] of Vedanta,[7] and *samkhya*,[8] which flows in the body of the Hindu tradition as philosophy and lifestyle. While playing, one automatically moves through different squares of the game board. Each square has a name, representative of an inner state as well as a plane. Each name triggers the mind and brings the consciousness of the player to contemplate and ponder the concept behind the word as long as he stays in that square. After a few minutes of playing, the game board starts to play with the mind and intellect of the player—as well as the ego, the strong sense of self-identity, the "isness" of the player.

---

*The explanations of the terms noted in this chapter begin on page 5.

Neither the author nor the date of origin of the game we now call Snakes and Arrows is known. As a general rule in the Indian literary tradition, the name of the author is considered unimportant. He is but a pen in the hands of God, a tool of expression; and so the name has not been recorded. The influences apparent in the formulation of the game point to an age of at least 2,000 years.

The copy used as the basis of this particular translation was preserved by the family of an author of commentaries, living in Uttar Pradesh about 150 years ago. The present author now has another older, but incomplete, copy of the game board in his possession, which he purchased in Rajasthan from an antique dealer. This copy is much older, but because it is not complete it was not used for writing this version of the commentaries.

A book of chants containing *schlokas*[9] accompanied the game board. With each toss of the die the player intoned the appropriate chant for the space in which he landed. The *schloka* described the nature and meaning of the space, represented by a square in the game board. Unfortunately, the book of chants has been lost, and it has become obligatory to write a commentary, showing the network of philosophical ideas indicated by the names of the squares and also introducing the method by which the game board can be used by those who are interested in knowing and playing the game. However, each Sanskrit term has a well-defined connotation within the context of the tradition from which the game sprang. In addition to these definitions, along with information obtained from saints (who played the game when they were young and when they joined their order) and the terminology used in the game board itself, some knowledge came to the author from his own family traditions. All this forms the basis of the present commentaries.

The creators of the game saw it foremost as a tool for understanding the relationship of the individual self to the Absolute Self. Played at this level, the game enables the player to detach himself from the illusion that his personality is firmly fixed. He sees his life as an expression of the macrocosm. Not his identifications but the play of cosmic forces determines the fall of the die, which in turn determines the course of his life's game. And the purpose of this game he sees as nothing less than the liberation of consciousness from the snares of the material world and its mergence with Cosmic Consciousness.

Just as one drop of water, taken from an ocean, contains all the elements present in the ocean that was its source, so too is human consciousness a microcosmic manifestation of Universal Consciousness. All that man can ever know already exists as a potential within himself. For all that man perceives is a product of his sensory organs.

Events in the phenomenal world trigger the five sensory organs (ears, skin, eyes, tongue, and nose). The affected sensory organ initiates in turn a biochemical process, which passes through the central nervous system to be manifested as variations in electrical activity in certain areas of the brain. This play of electrical energy is a gross manifestation of that aspect of consciousness called mind.

The mind presents sensory data to the intellect and ego for evaluation and action. It is from the sensory perceptions that all the desires arise. And desire is the essence of the game—the player would not play had he not the desire to play. Desires are the motivations of life: man lives to fulfill his desires.

Desires can be grouped in three classes, depending on their nature: physiological, sociological, and psychological. The physiological desires are those necessary for survival of the organism. Eating, drinking, sex, and sleep are major physiological desires. The sociological are physiological desires colored by the social context. Rather than one house, a man wants five. His need is for one, the desire for five—a social overlay. His desire for objects of luxury and a better status in society, which he can easily get by display of his achievements, is something that is social, and these desires are different in all parts of the world. Psychological desires all stem from the desire for identification of the self, the ego. The desire for inner growth and spiritual achievements is also a product of the ego. How strange it is that through this path one can lose the ego altogether: the great egotism of becoming egoless.

Physiological needs are recognized by all societies. No restrictions are placed on their fulfillment. Sociological desires vary from society to society. Psychological needs are common throughout the planet, and include man's complexes and achievements, disturbances and honors, enjoyments and traumas.

All these desires result from sensory perception and the faculty we call mind. All are biochemical states of the organism: all desires express themselves inside the organism as chemical states. As they produce chemical states, so can they also be provoked by the use of chemicals.

The physiological desires are often called animal needs, for they are the desires man has in common with all other animals. Psychological desires are often called higher needs, for they are concerned with the attachment of ego and the sense of fulfillment that comes from complete identification with the object of desire.

Whatever the source of the desire, the ego acts to fulfill it through five work organs (hands, feet, mouth, genitals, and anus). The action comes only after the sense perception, which was its source, has passed through the mechanisms of mind and intellect.

Each action triggers a reaction. The quality of the action determines the quality of the reaction. The reaction is manifested as a change in working consciousness. Negative actions entrap the player; positive actions liberate. "As ye sow, so shall ye reap": this paraphrase of a Biblical saying points out the law of karma.

Any action the player takes is proper as long as he realizes that all actions plant karmic seeds, which may not bear fruit for years. The fruits of karma may not even manifest in the present life but may submerge only to reappear in some future incarnation. It is these karmas from past lives that determine the course of personality development in the individual.

The real job of the player is to recognize these karmas and their effect on his being. From this awareness comes the knowledge required to raise his level of consciousness. This is the job of karma yoga.[10] And the phenomenal world is the stage on which the Leela (divine game) of karma is staged.

To understand the phenomenal world we must, then, become scientists of the self, exploring the organization of our own consciousness, the planes on which we dwindle all our lives, the snakes that we encounter, and the arrows we find in our upliftment. It is here the game of Leela serves its highest purpose. For it is a map of the self, the playground of the One-becoming-many.

Notes

1. Dharma: that which is inherent as law in the very nature of all existing phenomena, that which supports and holds the universe together. It is not merely a set of beliefs having no connection with living, but is rather a set of principles for a harmonious and beneficent life. It is a practical doctrine. The etymological meaning of dharma is also "that which binds together."

2. Vedas: divine knowledge, perfect knowledge, which is omnipresent and sustains all that is manifested. This knowledge is directly realized by rishis (saints, seers, yogis) through *samadhi*. This knowledge is available as four scriptures:
   a. Rig Veda.
   b. Yajur Veda.
   c. Sama Veda.
   d. Atharva Veda.

   Each Veda has three generally recognized divisions:
   a. Samhitas: collections of hymns or mantras.
   b. Brahmanas: containing precepts for establishing the mantras and ceremonies. They are treatises on rituals but are interwoven with many illustrative stories, philosophical observations, and profound ideas.
   c. Upanishads: philosophical treatises, based on interpretations given by rishis to whom this knowledge was revealed.

3. Shrutis: cosmic sound frequencies, floating in the cosmos as richis (incantations) revealed to rishis (visionaries). They contain the knowledge of the system by which the energies were vitalized in the universe at its beginning and are still directed by Cosmic Consciousness. Vedas are Shrutis.

4. Smiritis: practical application of divine knowledge and laws inherent in the

objects of the manifested universe. These treatises contain laws that make life divine. They are numerous, but four of them are very much quoted by scholars as the chief Smiritis:

    a. Manu Smiriti.

    b. Vagya Valka Smiriti.

    c. Shamkhya Smiriti.

    d. Parashara Smiriti.

Vedas are Shrutis, and all books dealing with the law of dharma are the Smiritis from which the basic structure of Hindu tradition was built by seers.

5. Puranas: next in order after Shrutis and Smiritis. They illustrate the philosophy of the Vedas through stories (from history) of those whose lives reflected the practical application of the law of dharma. They are allegorical in nature and explain the highest philosophy in a very human way. This is the reason the Puranas are called the fifth Veda.

6. Yoga: literally, to join, to unite, to add, union. It is a science of inner growth, which gives peace and the capability to stop mental fluctuations and modifications, which are the root cause of sufferings, miseries, and pain. It provides the ability to rise above the realm of the senses into habitual one-pointedness, undivided attention, perpetual peace, and enlightenment. It has numerous schools, which suggest and provide, each in its own way, methods for an overall development and growth of physical body and psyche (union of solar and lunar principles, control over the autonomic nervous system, etc.). Broadly it can be divided into three branches:

    a. *Karma* yoga: yoga of selfless action.

    b. *Gyana* yoga: yoga of cessation of mental modifications by negation, reaching the ultimate truth.

    c. *Bhakti* yoga: yoga of devotion, love, and surrender.

Famous schools of yoga include:

    a. *Raja* yoga: yoga of the eightfold path—*yama, niyama, asana, pranayam, pratiyahar, dharana, dhyana,* and *samadhi.*

    b. *Hatha* yoga: yoga that deals with the training of the senses by working with the body. It helps in achieving the goal designed by *raja* yoga.

    c. *Naad* yoga: yoga that deals with the sounds of the inner world.

      d. *Laya* yoga, and cosmic sound; also known as *kriya* yoga or *kundalini* yoga.

7. Vedanta: the philosophical doctrine, also. called Uttar Mimansa that dominates Indian thought to the present day, dealing with the nature of the self and discriminating between the real and unreal. It explains unity in diversity, the knowledge of noumena. It teaches one to climb from the idea of the individual self, which seems to be a reality apart from Cosmic Consciousness, to the thought that one is a part of the Supreme Self, the Brahman, and can unite with him; and finally that he is and ever has been the Cosmic Consciousness, veiled from himself by ignorance. Vedanta is the science of Self without attributes, and teaches "Thou art That."

8. *Samkhya:* the system of numbers; primarily an account of how creation started. It deals with the evolution of the manifested world.

9. *Schloka:* a Sanskrit verse.

10. Karma yoga: the yoga of selfless action (karma means action). Actions cover all acts done by the individual from birth to death. A player who performs karma with attachment uses any means that serve his purpose and in his selfishness causes harm to others. One who is not attached to his actions, and performs actions because they are unavoidable, performs karmas with a disinterested interest and does not adopt wrong means. Karmas performed by right means do not harm anybody and are in accordance with the law of dharma. Dharma is inherent in the player's own nature, if he performs karmas that coincide with the natural bent of his mind.

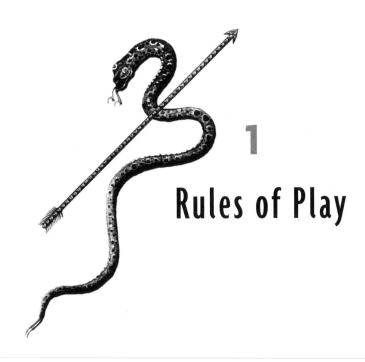

1
Rules of Play

Four things are necessary for playing Leela: the game board, a die (half a pair of dice), the commentary section of this book, and an object, such as a ring, that belongs to the player and is small enough to fit in the squares; this serves as the player's symbol during play. The rules are simple. Each player places his symbol in square 68, the square of Cosmic Consciousness. One by one, the players throw the die and pass it on to the player on the right (this conforms with the natural movement of upward-flowing energy).

The first player to throw a six moves to the first square, genesis, and from there to the sixth square, delusion. Until a six is thrown, the player must wait unborn in Cosmic Consciousness. Each time a six is thrown, at any stage in the game, the player rolls the die again. The exception to this is that a player who has rolled three sixes in a row (and has moved eighteen squares), and then rolls another number, must return to the place where he started before he began to throw the sixes, and move whatever number of squares is shown on the fourth roll. If, for example, a player throws three sixes and then another number on his fourth roll at the beginning of the game when his first six took him into play, he then returns to genesis (square 1) and counts forward the number shown on the fourth roll. But if, instead, he rolls four or more sixes, he continues to take additional turns until a number other than six is shown, at which point he moves the total number of squares he has thrown and passes the die.

When the player's symbol lands on the base of an arrow, he moves the symbol upward along the shaft of the arrow to its tip. If he lands on the head of a snake, it swallows him and deposits him at the tip of its tail. In this way, egotism leads to anger and spiritual devotion leads to Cosmic Consciousness. Thus the player throws the die and moves back and forth and up and down the board, taking care to move through the squares in ascending numerical order.

Returning to the sixty-eighth square is the object of play. If the player should reach the eighth level but pass by Cosmic Consciousness into the sixty-ninth, seventieth, or seventy-first square, he must wait to throw either the exact number required to land on *tamoguna,* the seventy-second square, or a lower number that would allow him to move one or two squares. From *rajoguna,* the seventy-first square, the throw of a one will return the player to earth, and back into the game. Play ends only when the player lands exactly on the sixty-eighth square, either by the arrow of spiritual devotion or by numerical ascension (such as being on square 66 and throwing a two).

In the course of play, the player will usually find that he has a characteristic pattern of landing on the same arrows and the same snakes. The game will take on its fullest meaning when the player reads and understands the commentaries, wherein are explained the meanings of each space, arrow, and snake.

If the player lands on square 69, the absolute plane, he cannot reach Cosmic Consciousness, which is square 68. In that case he has to reach square 72, where *tamoguna* can bring him back to earth, after which he can reach Cosmic Consciousness by gradual progression or by throwing a three and reaching spiritual devotion—the direct arrow to Cosmic Consciousness. While he is on square 69 he needs a three; on 70 he needs a two; on 71 he needs a one; all other numbers played by the karma die are useless, since he cannot make use of them any more than he can make use of a six when he is on 67. Throwing a one can bring him to 68, the place where the game stops, but the game continues if he throws a two, three, four, or five.

To have full advantage of the game, the player should note down the course adopted by the symbol that moves with the throw of the die on the game board. In a series of such recordings he would discover some common features: some friendly snakes and helpful arrows. This would compel him to find out the relationship between external and internal patterns. Saints have used this method to discover their inner pattern: it makes Leela, the yoga of snakes and arrows, a game of self-knowledge— "Gyan Chaupad."

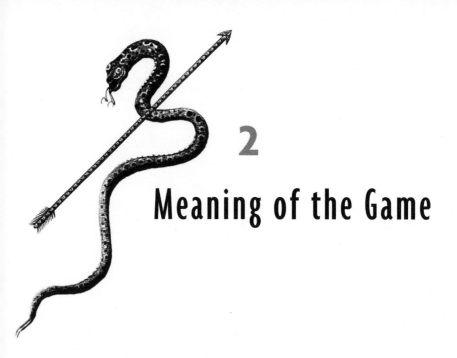

2

Meaning of the Game

Our perceptual world comes to us through the mechanisms of mind and intellect, which alter, color, and reject. Perceptions are received through organs that cannot perceive more than a millionth part of the total electromagnetic energy spectrum.

Thus the world that is known to us at any given moment is but one of an infinity of simultaneous events, any one of which could be perceived in an infinite number of ways because of the infinite number of possible organizations of mind and intellect. The possibilities are quite simply beyond comprehension.

Western science has specialized in the study of the sensory realm: the perceptual, phenomenal, material world. Its explorations have been carrying material science to a unifying point, a set of principles operating throughout the known cosmos. These principles transcend time and space. The light we receive from some galaxies is over 100,000,000 years old, yet it follows the same rules governing the light from our own sun, which is only nine light minutes distant.

These principles are expressed in formulas such as $E = mc^2$ and $3A^3$ (the organizing principle of every diamond in the universe). From diversity we are approaching a unity, expressed in the formulas of the physical sciences.

The Western mind has created a periodic table of the elements, which lists 103 fundamental organizations of matter. This is the essence of the West's understanding of the phenomenal world.

Eastern man, however, pursued a different course. In India, particularly, a temperate climate and the easy cultivation of crops did not force him to devote his energies to the struggle for survival that motivated the development of natural sciences in the West. Eastern man worshipped nature as a kind Mother principle and did not develop a conquest of nature that would prevent his own survival. The scientific spirit of Indian sages and seers turned inward to investigate the complexity that is human consciousness. Hence the science of tantra, yoga, and the ideas expressed in the Upanishads.

As general principles were discovered operating in the phenomenal world, so too were principles discovered in the operation of human consciousness. Yogis explored the labyrinth of the self and discovered seventy-two primary states of being. These states are the squares of the game of Leela, a periodic table of consciousness.

Within the seventy-two states, man acts out his karmic drama, play ending only when he attains total understanding of the game—Cosmic Consciousness. Play can be interrupted by the cessation of the principle of desire, but without a complete understanding of the game the true end of the game does not occur: desires are seeds of karma, and they can sprout any time they find suitable conditions to germinate. The player tosses his die, letting the forces of karma determine where he lands. He moves through the spaces and the various planes, up arrows and down snakes, until he is able to vibrate harmoniously everywhere, in all spaces. Ups and downs must lose their meaning.

The tossing of the die provides the variable link between the player's symbol and its movement across the game board. It is in the fall of the die that the principle known as synchronicity operates. Synchronicity is a term coined by the psychologist Carl Jung to explain the links that sometimes form between two seemingly unrelated events in the phenomenal world. Synchronicity is the fulfillment of a need by some agency outside the conscious control of the individual self. It is most easily understood in the context of interpersonal relationships. In a sense, synchronicity is being in the right place at the right time; and in reality, it is a continuous process.

In the game of Leela the need is understanding, the knowledge of how and where the player is experiencing at a given moment. The outside agency is karma, which determines the fall of the die. Leela is a game of synchronicity. Synchronicity simply means that all events in the phenomenal world are related and can be understood in their relationship if only a proper link can be forged. This game is such a link.

To strengthen the link, the player supplies an object of personal meaning to represent himself on the board. This is his symbol, and it moves across the board in accord with the tossing of the karma die. What is important is the pattern of movement of this symbol across the board. To understand this pattern—and the nature of the stages through which the player travels—it is necessary to understand more of the thinking on which the game board is based.

There is no death in this game. There are ups and downs, and changes in vibration levels, but there is no death. The spirit that is the individual self playing Leela does not die. It is the symbol, the body, moving across the game board with the toss of the karma die, which changes form. The individual self is a portion of the Lord, a limited manifestation of Cosmic Consciousness, the Supreme Self. The Divine dwells in the inmost being of man and cannot be extinguished. There is a vital unity of soul and body in man, as in the symbol and the player. The end only comes when the player reaches Cosmic Consciousness, the eternal state, the path from which there is no return. Here the player becomes the divine existence, beyond all modes and qualities. This is liberation. Death is change in form, not in spirit. It does not even exist on the material plane, because matter also is neither created nor destroyed but only changes form. Change of form is not real; it is a transitional phase in the world of phenomena, which is also an aspect of the Supreme, a reflexion of the Supreme Self. The cosmic process is an interaction between the two principles of Being and not-Being.

If we look at this game as a microcosm, we will find the complete octave of the macrocosm. As in a living organism the energy moves from plane to plane, from conception to birth, childhood to adolescence, youth to old age during a span of years, so the player operates from seven psychic energy centers moving up and down from chakra to chakra, and there are corresponding observable changes in his gross behavior.

Human life is a series of cycles: seven days for establishing conception, that is, for establishing the chemical nature; seven months to complete the formation of the body in the womb; and the seven major cycles of seven years each—the length of a complete lunar cycle—during which one moves through each of the psychic centers. In the game of Leela each of these seven cycles constitutes one horizontal row. The first center is the first row, and so on.

In the first cycle, to the age of seven, the player is too much himself—self-centered.

In the second cycle, seven to fourteen, he starts relating to a group of friends and living in the realm of fantasy. Attraction to the opposite sex, development of the aesthetic sense, and an interest in the fine arts also start at this age.

In the third cycle, fourteen to twenty-one, he wants to establish his identity. He wants power and affiliates himself to a group or ideology.

In the fourth cycle, twenty-one to twenty-eight, he begins to develop a sense of responsibility. He can now understand about others and appreciate their attributes.

In the fifth cycle, twenty-eight to thirty-five, he starts instructing others from his own experience and assumes the role of a teacher, often with the responsibilities of parenthood.

In the sixth cycle, thirty-five to forty-two, he becomes an observer of his own energy patterns and reviews his past karmas in the light of experience.

In the seventh cycle, forty-two to forty-nine, he is generally well settled and lives his life with the aim of finding and merging with truth.

This is the normal course of human development, but the environment into which the player is born dominates his pattern of thinking to a very high degree—and the karma die leads a player into the mouths of so many snakes of attachment that many people spend the whole of their lives on lower levels. There are others for whom all snakes seemingly vanish, and arrows magically appear to boost them to their goal in four or five moves.

The seven planes through which the player must pass before he reaches the eighth plane—the plane beyond all planes—are the seven chakras. Normally, energy would flow through these centers in a pattern synchronous with the vibrational rhythm of the player. During every twenty-four-hour period, life energy passes through all the seven chakras. At sunrise it is in the third chakra, and after sunset it comes to the seventh. Thus the energy is influenced by solar, lunar, and gravitational forces. But since few of us can live a pure and natural existence, complex blocks are formed in the energy pathways. It is not able to flow regularly and properly through the organism, creating a disparity between the mental and the chronological ages.

Each chakra has particular characteristics that enable the player to determine where he is vibrating at any given moment, particularly with the help of this game.

The first chakra is located at the base of the spine, midway between the anus and the genitals. Individuals vibrating here are insecure and are primarily concerned with physical survival. The sense of smell is dominant. The element of the first chakra is earth—the grossest manifestation of reality—and its color is yellow. The main problem of this chakra is violent behavior, which can arise from deep-rooted insecurity. However, the same insecurity can be a positive factor, as the motivating force behind the development of material technology. First-chakra people sleep ten to twelve hours nightly, on their stomachs.

The first chakra appears as the physical plane, the fifth square on the first row of the game. It is the plane of genesis, maya (the illusory perceptual world), anger, greed, delusion, conceit, avarice, and sensuality.

When a player enters into the game he has to pass through these nine squares. There are no arrows to lift him out of the first chakra, because these aspects of the first chakra are fundamental to human existence. If he does not feel concerned with society's value judgments, then he will know that all these things are important for human life. But if he is concerned with the world and its judgments, then he will say, "Well, anger is very bad. Greed is very bad. Vanity is very bad. All these things are very bad." They do create disharmony and bad body chemistry, increase selfishness, destroy inner peace, and so on, but as Shakespeare reminds us, "there is nothing either good or bad, but thinking makes it so." If we look deeper, from the point of view of survival (toward which first-chakra consciousness is oriented), we will see that without attachment, without greed, without a craving to find something more, life stagnates. If there were no anger and no vanity, the fun of the theater (Leela) would be lost. These various moods and temperaments provide color, the basic impetus for individual development. They are thought to be bad things, because they are connected with the lower, animal self. But we must see that they are also responsible for the growth and development of our rational, human, and divine self.

By mastering the first chakra the yogi obtains freedom from disease. By overcoming basic hang-ups he becomes open to knowledge, and no longer asserts himself so much. He learns to abstain from lower desires and attachments. Tantric scripture says he can become invisible if he wishes to.

In the second chakra, the player is caught up in the perception of his sensory organs. It is located in the region of the sex organs, with taste being its dominant sensory mode. Water is its element, and so it is characterized by luminous white or light blue. The principal problems associated with this chakra are corruption and disorder, ensuing from the loss of energy that comes from overindulgence in the sensory domain, and fantasy. But this same sensuality is the impelling force responsible for all the creative arts. One who vibrates in the second chakra sleeps eight to ten hours nightly in the fetal position.

The second chakra contains two arrows—purification and mercy—and two snakes—jealousy and envy. It contains the astral plane, the plane of fantasy, and the plane of joy. Here are found nullity and also entertainment, the essence of the spirit.

By mastering the second chakra the yogi becomes generally beloved. He can command the love of any animal or beast and can control the elements. He is freed from all his enemies and illuminates like the sun. He becomes well versed in prose, poetry, and reasoned discourse and can conquer lustful desires.

In the third chakra, the dominant characteristic is the recognition of the ego and a search for the immortality of the embodied being. As a fetus in the womb one receives nourishment to sustain development from this center. It contains the great junction of the right and left sympathetic chains with the cerebrospinal axis and is located at the root of the navel in the lumbar plexus, with connected sympathetic nerves concerned with the production of sleep and thirst. Sight is its dominant sensory mode. Fire is its element, and red the associated color.

The main problem of this chakra is exertion of power, imposing the will of the ego on others. The positive attribute is the organizational skill generated out of the altruistic use of power. One who vibrates here generally sleeps six to eight hours nightly on his back.

This third chakra is the celestial plane, and it contains three arrows—selfless service, dharma, and charity. There is one snake—bad company. It is the plane of sorrow, good company, atonement, and karma.

By mastering the third chakra one is able to destroy sorrow and disease and gain knowledge of different *lokas* (worlds). One develops the healing power. It is a chakra of stability, accumulation of power, accomplishment, command, control, and the worldly achievements necessary to ground one's ego.

In the fourth chakra the player becomes aware of karmas, the behavioral patterns of his life. He is vibrating from the heart region, the seat of the celestial wishing tree. The heart is the abode of the conscious principle—the life—and seat of *prana*. This chakra is the center of the seven: three are above and three below. Thus the heart chakra is influenced by higher and lower forces simultaneously. Air is the associated element, the color is smoky gray-green, and the sensory mode is tactile.

The main problem of the player here is a tendency toward imbalance, spending too much time trying to rectify that which was. Faith *(bhakti)* is the motivating force in his life. He sleeps on his left side, five to six hours nightly.

This is the plane of balance, and apt religion is the arrow that takes the player higher. The snake is irreligiosity, which takes the player back to delusion. Here are the planes of sanctity, fragrance, and taste. Here also are purgatory, good tendencies, and clarity of consciousness.

By mastering the fourth chakra the yogi becomes like Jupiter, the lord of speech. His senses are completely under control. He is dearer than the dearest to women. His life is inspired, and poetry flows in his speech like a stream of clear water—uninterrupted. Scriptures say he is able to transfer himself to another body. His very presence is inspiring, and he has no enemies. He gains the power to become invisible, and unnoticeable, and he can levitate at will. He is able to see objects of both the visible and invisible universes and has the ability to travel any part of the world by the exercise of his willpower. He gains mastery over time.

In the fifth chakra the player has realized compassion and wants to share with others how he has been able to resolve those karmas he has confronted. This chakra is located in the throat, at the junction of the spinal cord with the medulla oblongata. It is the chakra of *gyana* (also spelled *jnana*)—knowledge. The player becomes a knower, a *gyani* *(jnani)*. Without formal instruction and study he becomes knowledgeable of all scriptures *(shastras)*. He is constant, gentle, steady, modest, courageous, and free from diseases and sorrows. He is merciful toward everybody; he has no expectations. The main problem is authoritarianism: "This is the only way."

Beyond the realm of the senses, this chakra is the center of *akash* (ether). The elemental color is smoky purple. The player who vibrates here meditates on *soham* (*so* = that; *aham* = I am): "That I am"—the sound his breath makes as he inhales (*so* = sound of inhaling) and exhales (*ham* = sound of exhaling). His obsession is logic, and his boon understanding. His intellect becomes free from the impurity of worldly pursuits, and he can see past, present, and future within himself. Meditation upon the pit of his throat enables him to overcome hunger and thirst and to achieve steadiness. He sleeps four to five hours nightly, changing sides.

The fifth chakra is the human plane, and right knowledge and *gyana (jnana)* are the arrows that can take the player up. Ignorance is the snake. It is the plane of the positive, negative, and neutral life-breaths *(prana, apana, uyana)*. Here he is born as Man (a representative of higher consciousness as opposed to animal nature), and gains the understanding of energy, Agni (fire).

One who masters the fifth chakra can rejuvenate himself at will. His presence opens one to the knowledge of the Self, and in it one is able to understand the mysteries of nature and recognize the presence of divine knowledge in every existing phenomenon.

In the sixth chakra the dominant concern is *tapasya,* the austere task of raising consciousness ever higher. This is the center of command (*agya,* also spelled *ajna*) over movements. The player vibrating here has no problems. He is beyond seeing any possibility as a problem. He is centered in the third eye, the region of the pineal gland. He meditates on the sound *Om,* and on the sound of his breath, which he now hears as *hamsa* (*ham* = I am; *sa* = That) "I am That." There is a difference between *soham* and *hamsa.* In *soham* the yogi is in duality—he relates himself to the Supreme Consciousness, saying and feeling that That (Supreme Consciousness) I (individual consciousness) am. In the sixth chakra the duality dissolves, and undivided unity establishes itself in his consciousness. He is no more himself the individual, but he realizes that he is the Supreme Consciousness. He dwells in that union and meditates on his true nature. He is beyond the realm of the elements.

Conscience is the arrow here, and violence the snake. In this, the plane of austerity, we understand the operation of the solar, lunar, and neutral currents. *Pingala* and *ida,* which are the carriers of solar and lunar currents, come up to here from the *mooladhar* chakra and go to the nostrils, right and left, functioning with the breath. A carrier of neutral currents and *kundalini, sushumna* moves into the *Sahasrara.* From this plane, spiritual devotion—*bhakti*—can take the player directly to Cosmic Consciousness, the only direct path to liberation in the game, beyond both earth (the place of refuge) and the liquid plane (the plane of fluidity).

The player who masters this chakra obtains great psychic powers, and all karmas earned by him during different lives in the past are destroyed.

In the seventh chakra the player is beyond all pleasure and pain. He dwells in the thousand-petaled lotus at the crown of the head. Scriptures mention that one who establishes himself here in the seventh chakra becomes a master of eight *siddhis:* (1) *anima,* the power of becoming, (2) *mahima,* the power to enlarge, (3) *garima,* the power to become heavy, (4) *laghima,* the power to become light, (5) *prapti,* the power of reaching anywhere and everywhere, (6) *prakamya,* the power to realize all wishes, (7) *ishatva,* the power to create, and (8) *vashitva,* the power to command all. These powers, or *siddhis,* make him *siddha-purusha,* a real master, who by will can create anything. He does not become inert or inactive but is filled by the light of Supreme Consciousness and bliss.

But it is here that egotism can overtake him, and the *siddhis,* which are a great asset, can prove fetters; or inertia, *tamas,* can draw him down to illusion. On realizing the plane of reality he can experience positive and negative intellect—the latter a snake, which draws energy down to the second chakra. This is the plane of happiness, the gaseous plane, the plane of radiation, and the plane of primal vibrations.

The eighth horizontal row is beyond chakras. The seat of Cosmic Consciousness, it is the plane of the Absolute. Each of these nine squares is a God-force: the phenomenal world, inner space, bliss, and cosmic good. There are three phases of energy, which manifest with creation: (1) the dynamic/positive, (2) the inert/negative, and (3) equilibrium—*rajoguna, tamoguna,* and *sattoguna. Tamoguna* is responsible for evolution; *sattoguna* for dissolution or liberation. If Cosmic Consciousness is not realized, the player has to descend to earth to rejoin Leela until he achieves liberation by reaching and landing in Cosmic Consciousness. *Tamoguna* takes him back to earth, the playground of karma, where he must work his way back up from the sixth chakra.

Leela is the nature of Supreme Consciousness, the playful nature. The phenomenal world is manifested Leela. The play is beginningless as well as endless. Leela is the great adventure and the great discovery. Again, and again, and again, and again—without any loss, and without any gain—this endless game is played. Those who realize the *play* in the game are not caught by the game board and know it as the Leela (divine game) of Leela-Dhar (Cosmic Consciousness). Those who identify with the squares and planes of the game board are played by the game board; and the game board becomes maya, the great veiling power that binds the mind. It is maya that creates the phenomenal world. It is Leela that makes it a great adventure. *Tamas* brings the player to maya—and boundless love and spiritual devotion to Cosmic Consciousness. Spiritual devotion is the great discovery in the game board of Leela, created by maya of Supreme Consciousness in order to enjoy himself—to play hide and seek with himself. There is no purpose and no responsibility in Leela. In the words of Maharishi Raman:

> The ideas of purpose and responsibility are purely social in nature
> and are created by mind to exhort Ego. God is above all such ideas.

If God is immanent in all and there is no one except him, who is responsible for whom?

Creation is expression of inherent laws in the source of creation.

This inherent law is the playful nature of the Divine, which is Leela.

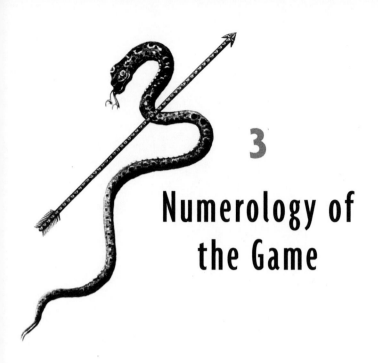

3

Numerology of the Game

The Indian tradition ascribes great significance to nine basic numbers, 1 to 9. Each number corresponds to a set of basic attributes, which contain keys to understanding the workings of the subtle life-force in gross manifestation. This is the teaching brought to the West by the Greek Pythagoras, a student of the Arabic version of Indian numerology.

In fact, not only do numbers count, but they give an account of the countless idea-forces working through human consciousness and the phenomenal world. They help the mind to have a definite idea of the perceptual world. In this beginningless creation there is neither first nor last, because all is one number. Actual digits are only the manifested forms, which appear as evolution starts and disappear or merge in their source with the dissolution of the phenomenal world. Everything that exists is disposed according to number, each a part *(ank)* of the whole (Brahman, Supreme Consciousness) manifesting himself. The whole is boundless, countless, no number, zero, *shoonya*—non-Being—which is the start of Leela, the cosmic play.

At the beginning is the separation of Being from non-Being. Sound, *naad,* is the first to evolve. Sound contains the twin aspects of sound and beat. Sound represents energy in its original vortex form. Beat is a pattern of vibration experienced in linear form. Sound creates space, and beat creates time. Each sound has a wavelength, and each wavelength exists in time. The measurement of a wavelength is the time that the wavelength takes from its origin to the end.

Plato regarded numbers as the essence of harmony and harmony as the basis of both cosmos and man. Balzac, the French novelist, called the numbers "incomprehensible agents." According to him, distinctions between different forms of existence are differences in their qualities, quantities, dimensions, forces, attributes, and nature. These differences are not in the essence, but in the material content, which is arranged in different patterns. These patterns, when observed closely, vary only in numbers. The difference between an atom of copper and one of gold is but a difference in the number of particles they contain.

72	71	70	69	68	67	66	65	64
55	56	57	58	59	60	61	62	63
54	53	52	51	50	49	48	47	46
37	38	39	40	41	42	43	44	45
36	35	34	33	32	31	30	29	28
19	20	21	22	23	24	25	26	27
18	17	16	15	14	13	12	11	10
1	2	3	4	5	6	7	8	9

The arrangement of the playing board of Leela is based on a foundation stone of numerology. The board is a numerologically balanced perfect rectangle. It contains eight horizontal rows from bottom to top. Eight is the number of the manifested universe, *prakriti,* which is composed of the five elements, or *mahabhutas* (ether, air, fire, water, and earth) and the three forces—mind, intellect, and ego *(manas, buddhi, ahamkar)*. The vertical columns from left to right total 9, the number of the Absolute, Supreme Consciousness (the eight of *prakriti* plus one—Consciousness). Nine is the completion of the series of simple (basic) numbers and is therefore the number of completion. Thus there are seventy-two squares making up the field of cosmic play. Seventy-two when reduced to a simple whole number again becomes 9 (7 + 2 = 9).

In the serpentine motion of play, the start of each horizontal column begins with a number reducible to 1 and ends on a number that reduces to 9. For example, the second horizontal row begins with 10 (1 + 0 = 1) and ends on 18 (1 + 8 = 9). In addition, each horizontal row contains nine numbers, which when added together yield the number 9. The first row totals 45 (4 + 5 = 9), the second 126 (1 + 2 + 6 = 9), the third 207 (2 + 0 + 7 = 9).

Each vertical column, except the central one, contains just two basic numbers. The first column consists of 18 (1 + 8 = 9), 19 (1 + 9 = 10 = 1), 36 (= 9), 37 (= 1), 54 (= 9), 55 (= 1), and 72 (= 9). The second vertical column yields 2s and 8s, the third 3s and 7s, the fourth 4s and 6s, and the fifth the only exception—all 5s. From here the order reverses (6s and 4s, 7s and 3s, 8s and 2s). So each vertical column, except for the middle, contains two fundamental integers, which when added together produce 1. The central column, the column of balance, contains 5s; and two 5s yield 10 or 1. In addition, the sum of each vertical column is 292, which becomes 4 (2 + 9 + 2 = 13 = 1 + 3 = 4), the number of rational organization, tangible achievement, tetramorphs, the formless square.

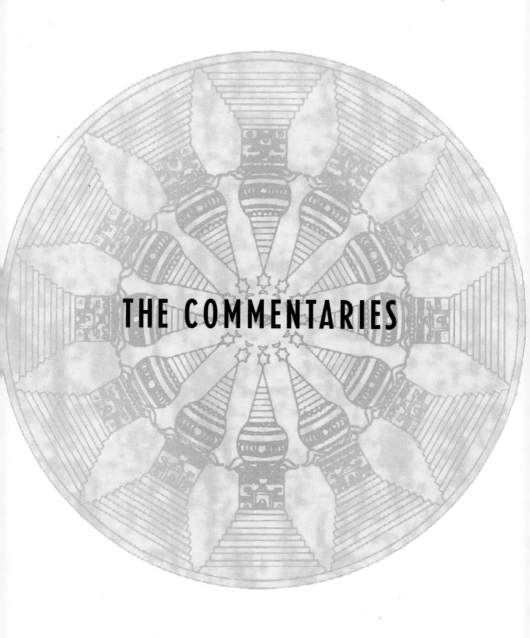

THE COMMENTARIES

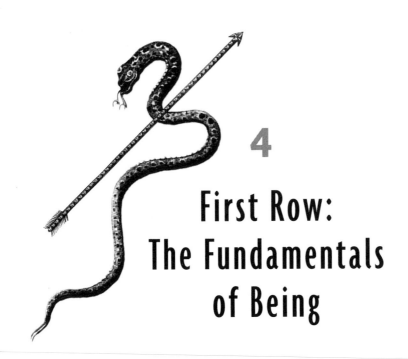

4

First Row:
The Fundamentals
of Being

1

Genesis
(janma)

Birth is entry into the karmic play. The die is the karmic player, and the individual self a symbol that moves from house to house, wherever the die determines. Before taking birth one is beyond the game. Once birth is taken, one is bound by the law of karma. This world is karmaland.

Desire leads the player to accept the bondage of karma. If one has no desire to play, one will not be attracted toward the game. But play is in the nature of consciousness. In the beginning there was no play; but the playful nature of consciousness could not remain motionless, without playing. So . . . "Let there be light." Let there be play. The Absolute became many from One, to play the game.

When the player decides to enter the game he is re-enacting the primordial creation, when the Absolute stirred from inaction and began the macrocosmic play in which we are all but microcosms. Once the decision to play is made, the player must abide by the rules (dharma), the bondage of the karma die.

It is here that the player first enters into the game after throwing a six. When the five subtle elements (ether, air, fire, water, and earth) and one consciousness unite, these six initiate the movement of the player's symbol across the board. Each birth is the opening of a new game, and the object of attainment in each game is the same Cosmic Consciousness. There is no other directive, no other goal, no other purpose in playing the game. The game is just to complete the cycle. Birth is the key. It opens the doors of the game, and the player begins to vibrate as he starts on the eternal voyage, his journey toward completion.

One is the unity responsible for all manifestation. Like all odd numbers it belongs to the sun family. One especially denotes the sun, which is the unity responsible for the birth of this planet. One represents independent personality, independent decision, independent life, the search for something new, novelty, originality.

2
Illusion
(maya)

When one accepts entry into the game as a player, awareness of unity is lost in the obsession (fascination) of play. This taking over of consciousness is the fun of play. The One becomes many, to play a game of cosmic hide-and-seek with itself. To fulfill his ego, the player sets up the game and its rules and commits himself to playing them out to the end.

The One is reality. Multiplicity is illusion. This illusion of multiplicity is created by the veiling power of the One (the Supreme Consciousness). This veiling power is called Maya Shakti, or maya. This veiling power creates the illusion of *me* and *mine,* or *thee* and *thine,* which creates ignorance in the individual consciousness. Those who

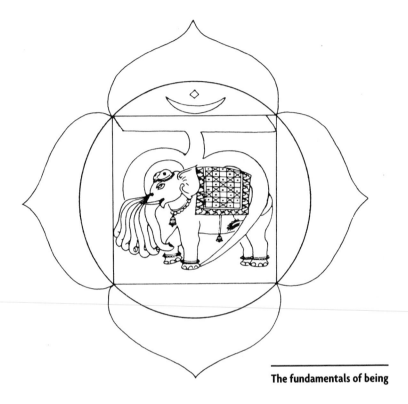

The fundamentals of being

realize this ignorance call it *avidya* (*a* = no; *vidya* = knowledge; thus ignorance, or absence of knowledge). So maya is also called *avidya* by yogis. This ignorance comes to individual consciousness through the mind; that is why yoga is a practical device to stop the modifications of mind, and yoga's aim is to arrest mind, to stop the inner dialogue, to go beyond the mind and realize one's true nature, beyond the illusion of *me* and *mine*.

The world of names and forms is maya. Maya is the stage and setting within which the player enacts his microcosmic tragicomedy. Maya is the play itself, presenting the player with situations and patterns that offer him subtle clues to the understanding of his own true nature.

This illusion can be seen at every level. The human body itself is not a unit of existence, but is composed of countless numbers of cells and micelles. If each cell starts growing a sense of *me* and *mine*, each human body will become a subcontinent. It is the individual ego *(aham-kara)* that creates separate units of existence—but this in itself is maya (illusion). Ego cannot function without mind, as mind cannot without sensory organs. So it is only after the mind is brought to a suppressed state that the sense of *me* and *mine* can be completely annihilated. By yoga alone can this state be achieved and an end brought to this illusory sense of being an independent unit. After realization of truth through a direct experience of reality in *samadhi,* Maya Shakti can be understood and the human psycho-drama can be observed as divine play, as Leela.

Maya Shakti is the power that brings forth the evolution of the phenomenal world. It makes this possible by an interplay of the three *gunas: sattva, rajas,* and *tamas.*

Cosmic Consciousness becomes individual consciousness by its own maya. In Hindu literature maya has been described in very many contexts, and yet it is impossible to explain all about it—it is as infinite as Cosmic Consciousness itself.

The only job confronting the player is the realization that he is a player, that the sense of separation he feels is illusory. All that the player perceives of the phenomenal world exists within himself in the form of sensory input and is illusory. Modern sciences that try to investigate the nature of truth verify this statement. Both modern science and ancient wisdom believe in a single primordial substance to which the various forms of matter can be reduced. All phenomenal existence is but one of the many manifestations of the same underlying unity. The elements are varied forms of this one substance. The variety of our experience is due to the permutation and combination of atoms of the matter into which this primordial energy materializes. This diversity in unity is illusion and is caused by the veiling power of the Supreme Consciousness. All that the player perceives of the phenomenal world exists within himself. One takes birth to play the game, to discern the subtle principles at work within the gross. The game is to reach unity, to end duality.

The number 2 signifies duality, which is illusion. Two comes into being when 1 repeats itself. Two is maya, because both were present in the One. The two are the internal and the external world; the unmanifested and the manifested, Shiva and Shakti, male and female, sun and moon, gross and subtle, Absolute and maya, noumenon and phenomenon. Two is therefore the number of maya. Two is an even number and, in common with all even numbers, is a member of the moon family; it is especially related to the moon and lunar energy.

3

Anger
(krodh)

An understanding of the nature of ego is essential to the comprehension of anger. The ego is that which identifies itself as *me* and *mine*. Man is a being who grows through a process of successive identifications. After taking birth, the child first identifies himself as a separate being when he begins to sense separation from his mother. Next comes identification with the other members of his family, adopting their behavior patterns and thought forms as his own. Then the child begins to associate with peers of the same sex. Later in life he seeks his identity in members of the opposite sex.

The end of his journey comes when his ego makes its final identification with the Absolute and merges into Cosmic Consciousness.

Ego works with intellect in the identification process. The intellect stores the information received in the identification process, especially the value judgments received from those with whom the being identifies most closely. The real Self within knows that all realities are contained within itself. However, the identifying self excludes these aspects adjudged evil by those with whom it identifies.

Anger is the emotional/chemical reaction produced when the ego is confronted with an aspect of self that it has rejected and judged as evil. The existence of this negative aspect is experienced as a threat to existence. Indeed, the existence of the current self-identification does face a genuine threat. The ego then projects the rejected aspect of self onto the other through whom it is manifested, and directs its energy toward removing the undesirable aspect. This is the nature of anger.

Anger is a manifestation of multiplicity, of weakness. It is the tail of the snake of egotism. It is a downward projection of energy, which brings the player to the first chakra. When the ego is hurt one feels anger. Anger is insecurity—the basic first-chakra obsession.

Anger is a great obstacle in the path of spiritual growth. It produces fire and heat, and burns everything. But whenever this anger is produced without any personal feelings, and is impersonal, it purifies. Anger is a quality of Rudra, the lord of destruction. His anger is not based on personal reasons, and so it destroys not him but the evil that causes disharmony and disbalance. Anger aroused by personal reasons eats the gentle qualities of the self, and brings energy down. Anger aroused by impersonal reasons destroys its own cause, which is evil. Anger is the other side of love. We cannot be angry with those with whom we do not identify. Anger excites the nervous system and suspends the rational mind completely for the time it stays with the system. In one way it purifies the body and is very similar to fire-cleaning, but the cost is too high because it brings a person too low, and he has to start once again from the first row of the game.

Anger can be expressed in two ways: violence or nonviolence. When nonviolence is adopted as a means of expressing anger, it creates great moral strength and becomes *satyagrah* (*satya* = truth; *agrah* = persistence). This is possible only when the player remains calm, even though he really is experiencing anger. This anger is impersonal. It is against evil. It is based on love: love of good, love of truth. This anger helps spiritual growth and is divine.

Three is the number of creativity, expression, and stability. A member of the family of odd numbers, 3 is dynamic, and positive; it establishes a pattern. It signifies the fire element, which in human beings is manifested as anger. On the positive side, the same element can become zeal. Thus power and determination are characteristics of number 3. Three is the number of the planet Jupiter. Jupiter is a symbol of boldness, courage, power, strength, labor, energy, knowledge, wisdom, and spirituality.

4

Greed

(lobh)

The feeling of separateness brought about by taking birth creates a craving for fulfillment. In order to function in the world, the player must first make certain his physical needs are met. In order to join the game the player must eat, have a place to rest, and have clothing to wear. Material survival is the primary concern in the first chakra.

Greed arises when the player confuses his sense of unfulfillment with the need for material survival. Having attained the basic necessities of life, he still feels empty. All he has learned is how to maintain his physical existence. So he employs these basic survival skills to acquire more and more material belongings in the hope of fulfilling himself.

The more he acquires, the deeper his compulsion becomes. His sense of emptiness reaches the level of panic as his actions become increasingly desperate. The legend of King Midas and his touch of gold is a classic Western tale of the consequences of greed. This craving for material success is also the root cause of all military conquest.

Greed comes from insecurity, and insecurity from misidentification of Self. When a player does not believe in God, he does not believe in providence. Greed is the tail-end of the snake of jealousy. Greed makes a player short-sighted. He does not realize that greed is ultimately pointless. In the end, all material possessions are left behind, whether willingly or by the intercession of death. But greed can prove an asset in spiritual growth if one becomes greedy for spiritual experiences, knowledge, and love.

The player who falls into greed also opens the gates to maya, anger, and all other first-chakra problems.

Four is symbolized as a square representing the four dimensions, the four directions. It symbolizes the earth element. As a member of the family of even numbers, 4 tends toward completion. The impetus for completion, carried to its extreme on the material plane, becomes greed. In numerology, the number 4 is ruled by *rahu*, the north node of the moon, also known as the Dragon's Head. In western numerology, 4 is ruled by Uranus. In occultism, it is always written as 4–1 and as such is considered to be related to the sun as well.

5
Physical plane
(bhu-loka)

A portion of unmanifested reality transforms itself into the world of names and forms. The world of names and forms exists in seven different *lokas,* or levels, which exist in an ascending scale.

These *lokas* mark the stages of evolution of the consciousness of the individual. As he evolves, so he moves and undergoes modifications in his nature. Through these planes the consciousness is able to realize its true nature.

Each of these *lokas,* or planes, is a definite region, marked off by the nature of the matter of which it is composed. (See square 32, plane of balance.)

These *lokas* form the spine of the game board. They are all in their definite order in the central row of vertical squares.

As it is in the macrocosm, so is it in the microcosm. The *lokas* are located in the human body along the spine, at the chakras, the psychic centers. With the evolution in the psyche from level to level comes evolution in the man himself.

The physical plane is located at the base of the spine, the site of the first chakra in the human body—and on earth in the phenomenal world. The name *bhu-loka* in Sanskrit explains it: *bhu* means earth and *loka* means plane. Earth is made of five elements, which exist in solid, liquid, and gaseous forms—as radiant, etheric, and superetheric matter—the various stages of existence of atoms of matter, whether defined as form or undefined. The earth element, under all conditions in all circumstances, is dominant in them, and they materialize as earth slowly and gradually.

Other planes mentioned in the game board each fall in a certain horizontal row and belong to these seven *lokas*. The *lokas*, other than the seven seated in the spine of the game board, are special regions situated within the seven—like cities in provinces, provinces in countries, and countries in continents.

The physical plane encompasses genesis, maya, anger, greed, delusion, conceit, avarice, and the sensual plane—its right and left sides, its positive and negative aspects.

When the player moves on to the physical plane he becomes trapped by the lower self. This is just one phase of the game. No one stays in the same place all the time. Each throw of the die is an opening to a new world.

On the physical plane the player is mostly concerned with material achievements. Money, house, vehicle, food, and physical power are common themes. His recreation is bodily involvement, sports involving competition and physical contact. His fun can too often include violence. His major achievement is craft.

The physical plane is related to earth, matter, and mother. It is the storehouse of energy, the dwelling place of *kundalini*—the psychic energy the yogi seeks to raise up through the seven chakras. Without realization of the physical plane, realization of all other planes is impossible. There are no arrows leading from this plane, this horizontal level. All players must pass through it before reaching the other dimensions. Seven snakes lead here from other planes, demonstrating the primary importance of realizing the nature of the grossest level of manifestation.

The number of subtle elements is five—ether, air, fire, water, and earth. Five also are the work organs man employs in the creation of karmas—hands, feet, mouth, genitals, and anus. And there are five sensory organs for five sensations—ears for sound, skin for touch, eyes for sight of form and color, tongue for taste, and nose for smell. Five is the number of balance—1 with 2 on each side. The ruling planet of number 5 is Mercury. Mercury is gentle, the high thinker, scholar, and lover of entertainment, and also is connected with business and physical comforts.

6
Delusion
(moha)

Moha in Sanskrit means attachment. This attachment is the real cause of bondage, bringing the player time and again to the phenomenal world through a series of births and rebirths. It is said in scriptures that four obsessions lead the individual consciousness into a downward flow of energy; they are obstacles in spiritual growth. These four are called

> *Kama:* desires, sensuality
> *Krodh:* anger, aggression, violence
> *Lobh:* greed, dissatisfaction
> *Moha:* attachment, delusion

While illusion, maya, is the phenomenal world itself, delusion is attachment to the phenomenal as the only possible manifestation of reality. Delusion beclouds the mind, rendering it unfit to perceive truth. Delusion is the product of irreligiosity—religion meaning here not a code of conduct and morals (ethics) but a life lived in harmony with the laws of the universe.

"Whatever should be adopted, that is dharma," advises an old Sanskrit saying. Dharma is the nature, the essence, the truth of phenomenal existence. When a player does not follow the law of his own nature, which is beyond all illusion and delusion, he becomes mired in delusion. One has but to understand that existence is a game. With this realization, the delusion of being a self-directed player vanishes. And with the disappearance of the delusion, bad karma too vanishes.

Delusion is the first square on which the player lands after throwing the six he needs to enter the game. In entering play, the player accepts temporary bondage to the material realm. After the player is born, he is conditioned to accept the particular circumstances of time and place as binding. The reality of the moment is perceived as the reality of all moments. Change is inconceivable. He has fallen into delusion.

However he gets here, by taking birth or by falling prey to the snake of irreligiosity (the use of bad means, selfish measures), the player inevitably passes through delusion. Once he sees his dharma and recognizes that change is not only possible but necessary, he is ready to move on. But as long as he sees his own way of perceiving the world as closed and complete, he is destined to return here again and again.

Because of its nature as a combination of two odd numbers and two even numbers (two 3s and three 2s, or five combinations of pairs), 6 is a perfectly balanced number. Related to inventiveness, creativity, and the fine arts, six is a moon-family member and is associated with the planet Venus. Venus is the most shining and brilliant of all the planets and can be seen by the naked eye as the morning star. In Hindu mythology, Venus is the teacher of demons. Those who dwell in delusion love sensual pleasures, spend their energy in the fulfillment of desires, are victims of anger and greed, act against the law of dharma, and are irreligious and extremely selfish.

7

Conceit

(mada)

Conceit is self-deception, false pride, building castles in the air. The word *mada* in Sanskrit means self-intoxication. The player is intoxicated by false vanity, pride, power, possessions, accomplishments, or achievements. When he has any kind of delusion about himself, he is taken over by *mada*.

After entry into the game the player becomes subject to *mada,* conceit, false identification of all kinds. Pride and vanity are two great intoxicants—and one drinks them in bad company. Bad company, the outcome of delusion and greed, is the snake that leads the player to conceit. In this space the player is completely trapped by his own game. The bad company he keeps is a manifestation of evil desires.

Everyone plays his own game and throws his own die. Once the die is cast he has no option. A player with no desires does not seek out company. But since desire is in the nature of the game, the seeking out of company is inevitable at some point in his development. The player needs a group to reinforce new identifications. The danger comes when the player is overwhelmed by his desires. His behavior patterns alter radically. The right no longer seems right, nor the wrong improper. His desire must be sated at any cost, and thus he creates bad karmas and keeps bad company—those who support him in his wrongdoing. As a man is known by the company he keeps, the player can stop generating bad karmas by seeking out good company.

A sun-family member, 7 is associated with Saturn and the principle of darkness. Seven are the days, the notes of the musical scale, the days of the week, and the chakras. One with two odd numbers (two 3s) on either side, seven is the number of the problems of adjustment. Seven is lonely in nature, and aspires for completion.

Seven is associated with *ketu,* the south node of the moon, also known as the dragon's tail. In modern Indian numerology, the number 7 is ruled by Varuna, the deity presiding over water, which is related to the planet Neptune in Western numerology. Seven is the number of writers and painters, who, when not evolved, live in false pride and are famous for building castles in the air and being always anxious about the future. They dislike following the beaten track and have very peculiar ideas about religion. They create a religion of their own and spend their life in amusement.

8

Avarice

(matsar or *matsarya)*

Conceit leads the player to feel envious of others. He is so obsessed with the delusion of being a separate reality that no means of fulfilling his desire seems unjustifiable. After all, thinks the conceited player, I am so much better than others that I deserve what they have. So in this game avarice is linked with the snake of envy—for it is the envy created by conceit that leads to avarice.

In the state of avarice the player has an active dislike of other players. He is too good for them, and what they have is also too good for them. Therefore, he reasons, what they have should be his. He becomes spiteful and lusts after the material belongings of his fellows. This contrasts with greed, where only the material is seen. Avarice is greed coupled with envy. As he becomes more avaricious his thirst for wealth increases, and all the other first-chakra problems begin to plague him.

Eight is a number that decreases when multiplied: $8 \times 1 = 8$; $8 \times 2 = 16 = 1 + 6 = 7$; $8 \times 3 = 24 = 6$; $8 \times 4 = 32 = 5$; $8 \times 5 = 40 = 4$; $8 \times 6 = 48 = 3$; $8 \times 7 = 56 = 2$; $8 \times 8 = 64 = 1$. When eight realizes 9—thus $8 \times 9 = 72$—it becomes 9, and on the next cycle it returns to its original state, $8 \times 10 = 80 = 8$. This phenomenon is synonymous with the cyclical nature of all reality and the process of human existence. The subtle diminishes as the gross increases, until the heart of the gross is penetrated and becomes subtle again. Thus every increase decreases; every decrease increases. Nothing is ever lost. Only the nature of manifestation changes.

Among the moon-family numbers, 8 represents the octave, the eight dimensions, the eightfold maya (three *gunas* and the five subtle elements). In numerology, 8 is the moon's north node, and it is associated with the planet Saturn. This is a complex planet, difficult to understand. It has many ups and downs, and terrible struggles. It is an "airy" planet, associated with darkness, and is symbolized as a silent thinker or a servant, introspective and materialistically minded. People born under the number 8 collect wealth as a hobby and are subject to addiction and vice. But they are wise and experienced and have a special ability to judge people.

9

Sensual plane
(kama-loka)

This is the ninth square of the first row. Nine is a complete number, an odd number, and marks the completion of the first row. It is a ladder leading to the second level of consciousness, which begins with purification. After taking birth into the game, the player has to pass through the sensual plane before he can enter into the second level.

Kama in Sanskrit means desire, desire of any kind and every kind— for name, fame, wealth, success, family, position, accomplishment. Any kind of desire, ambition, or noble or nonnoble aim is *kama*. And *kama* is the first stage in evolution. If there were no desire there would not be any creation.

So *kama-loka* is a plane of desires. But since all desires have their origin in man's sensual nature, this is known as the sensual plane. It is directly linked with ignorance, the lack of knowledge. One may come here through the mouth of the snake of ignorance or through the gradual exploration of the first chakra. Nine, a member of the family of odd numbers, signifies completion and perfection. It represents force and energy. Multiplied by any other number, it retains its identity and integrity; thus: $9 \times 1 = 9$; $9 \times 2 = 18 = 1 + 8 = 9$; $9 \times 3 = 27 = 9$; $9 \times 4 = 36 = 9$; and $9 \times 23 = 207 = 9$; $9 \times 376 = 3,384 = 9$; $9 \times 280 = 7,380 = 9$. There are nine gates of the body through which the vital energy, *prana,* leaves at the time of death: the mouth, the two nostrils, the two eyes, the two ears, the anus, and the sex organ. During a day of twenty-four hours a man breathes 21,600 times, which reduces to 9. The day contains 1,440 minutes, also reducing to 9. The normal duration of the dominance of one hemisphere or one nostril is about 900 breaths (60 × 15), reducing to 9. There are nine major nerves of the body. Nine goddesses, *navdurgas,* are worshipped in Hindu religion. There are 72,000 nerves in the body, called *nadis.* These are carriers of *prana,* the vital life-force, and their total also reduces to 9. There are nine planets in the solar system influencing life on planet earth, known as *Navgrahas.* In numerology 9 is the number of Mars, which shines in the sky with a beautiful red glitter.

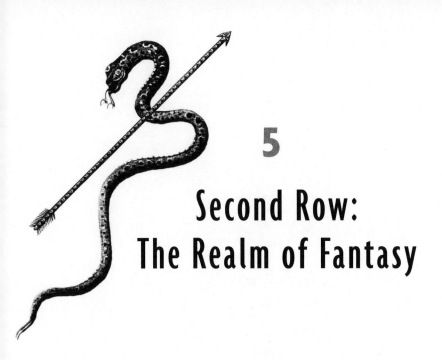

5

Second Row:
The Realm of Fantasy

10
Purification
(shuddhi)

For a time, the player feels comfortable on the sensual plane. But soon the downward flow saps his vital energy, leaving behind feelings of emptiness and confusion. At this moment purification draws his attention. Purification is the first arrow of the game and provides the opportunity to transcend all second-chakra problems. If after passing through the first chakra he lands on purification, the player purifies himself of all first- and second-chakra problems and rises immediately to the celestial plane.

Purification always refers to an increase in the vibrational level of the being, which causes energy to flow in an upward direction. Purification can be achieved through altering the behavior of the sensory organs, the work-organs, and the normal pattern of daily existence. There are five windows in the castle of consciousness. Through these windows, the enemies (impurities) enter into the castle and attempt to destroy the

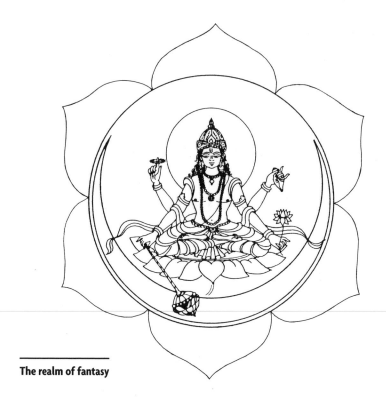

The realm of fantasy

king. By closing these windows, or by maintaining a proper watch, the player can keep the castle pure.

Purification of the ears is accomplished by withdrawing the power of hearing from the outside and attending to inner sounds. Purification of the eyes comes when they are closed, and all attention is focused on the third eye, at the center of the forehead just above the brow line. Purification of the tongue, the window of taste, can be attained by eliminating sweet and salty tastes from the diet. Purification of smell is done through closing the nostrils and retaining the breath in the lungs for as long as possible (this also helps develop the habit of deep, slow breathing). Rubbing ashes on the skin purifies the sense of touch, making the player immune to sensations from the epidermal nerves.

Through the process of sleep-fasting—going without sleep day and night for one day or several—the player can purify himself of inertia, dullness, drowsiness, stupidity, and ignorance. By speech-fasting—going without uttering a sound for extended periods—the thought process becomes purified. Food-fasting purifies the body chemistry. In addition, going through hardships purifies the player's personality, listening to scriptures and divinely inspired poetry purifies his inner self, humming purifies his nerves, and concentration and meditation purify both mind and body. Celibacy also is one of the methods of purification, a hard but very effective way of changing the vibrational pattern.

11

Entertainment
(gandharvas)

It is said in scriptures that *gandharvas* are "His" musical notes. The word *gandharvas* in English can be translated as celestial musicians. They come under the eight kinds of creation that cannot be perceived by the normal eye; but they have the power to adopt a form at will. They are not composed of gross material particles, for they dwell on the astral plane. Their wives are called *apsaras* (nymphs), and together in every manner they entertain God and those who have by their evolution reached this plane. They have surrendered themselves for the entertainment of the gods of the celestial plane. As celestial musicians they live in harmony with divine music. In the stories of the Puranas there are numerous references to the acts of *gandharvas* and *apsaras*. They are initially free from the cycle of birth and death—but if they do not act in harmony with their state of being, they fall to earth from heaven, and take birth as human beings. But wherever they exist, they provide entertainment.

The player enters into the state of entertainment after purification. This space is an expression of inward joy, a feeling of rhythm, a sense of harmony. Entertainment makes him light and provides the incentive for recreation and amusement. Entertainment brightens mundane existence and provides new avenues, new vistas, new horizons. All the fine arts are a product of this state, which belongs to the second row of the game and is an attribute of vibration in the second chakra. But entertainment exists at all levels. This game board, Leela or Gyan Chaupad, is an entertainment for the saints.

Life is based on the principle of entertainment—fun. And life can be perceived as entertainment when the player has transcended the level of the first chakra (security). The essence of spirit is entertainment. The whole of the creation is an entertainment of energy—by Shakti, the mother principle, the Absolute, God . . . or whatever the Supreme Player, who playeth not, may be called. If the Divine Play (entertainment) were not itself involved in the game, then the One would not choose to become many. It is in the process of entertainment that the One becomes many. To entertain is to accept. To accept is to surrender. And to surrender is to dissolve and become One.

12

Envy
(eirsha)

Envy is the first snake of the game. Its bite brings the player down from the second chakra to avarice and to all else that comes with vibrating in the first chakra. Time and again this little snake catches the player and brings him down. When he lands in envy he feels a lack of confidence in himself and resorts to first-chakra strategies for overpowering his desire. In the process of the game, this serpent helps the player to purify his thought process.

In the game of life, energy moves from below to above. The player wants to leave the lower planes and reach the summit, forever abandoning the problems he encountered below. But this attitude runs contrary to the very essence of the game. He has to play in all the planes, below and above—wherever his karma die leads him.

But nobody wants to remain low. When the player does not vibrate correctly the snakes get hold of him. And by his own throw of the die the player comes and goes, up and down. Envy is felt when the energy is down. The player has only by karmic chance reached a higher plane and really does not deserve to stay there. He cannot, in fact, remain there, because negative vibrations are still present in his being. At such times he feels envious of those he sees who are able to remain steadily on the higher planes. This envy is a negative reaction, which draws his energy back down to the first chakra, where he must work out more karmas.

13

Nullity

(antariksha)

Antariksha is the space between the physical plane, which is earth, and the celestial plane, *swarga,* which is heaven, the kingdom of God. This space is neither on earth nor in heaven, it is between the two planes. Neither here nor there, no-where: nullity.

Nullity is a state directly linked with the unstable negative intellect. When a player lacks awareness of the purpose of his being, feelings of meaninglessness (existential *angst*) and futility flow through his consciousness. He has no sense of purpose, leading him to seek out the company of his fellows. But the lack of vital energy creates such feelings of futility that he does not stay in any one place, though he dwells continually in negativity.

Nullity is a manifestation of the second chakra and the cause of inactivity, instability, and restlessness. Everything loses meaning. Nothing excites. The identification of personality is completely lost, resulting in an imbalance of the mental state. All this happens because the player lacks the energy necessary to function in the higher planes. The depletion of energy in the pursuit of sensory objects is the fundamental trap of the second chakra. The player may land in nullity after first hitting entertainment, the sensual plane, conceit, or avarice. If he comes here from the first chakra he has experienced the joys of purification and entertainment but has expended his limited energy too rapidly. Now he is confused. The goals he saw before are still there, but what is the use? What use is anything?

But nullity is not a permanent state, and soon he begins to regain his energies. He is ready to play again by the time the die comes around.

14

Astral plane
(bhuvar-loka)

Bhuvar-loka, the plane next to the physical plane, is closely related to it but composed of finer matter. We have already explained (in the description of *bhu-loka*, the fifth square of the first row of the game board) the presence of seven *lokas* and have explained that each *loka* is a state of being in the process of inner growth, the grossest being the physical plane *(bhu-loka)*. In *bhuvar-loka* the water element is predominant, as it is in the second chakra. As the second chakra is situated in the spine adjacent to the first chakra, so is the astral plane directly above the physical plane in the spine of the game board.

This is the plane of dreams and fantasy, where the human imagination begins to soar. The player who lands here becomes aware of the immense diversity of the phenomenal world. The world literally comes alive with possibilities. There are so many things he can be, so many goals he can pursue. This awareness of possibilities creates excitement, and he begins to take a more active interest in life. He has met his survival needs, and now he sees that there is far more to life than he could ever have imagined while he was still worried about where his next meal would come from.

Now he is materially secure, and his success is assured. And with this surge of self-reliance his creative imagination takes flight. But fantasies consume more energy than any other human activity. The player diverts his entire energy resources to building castles in the air. He strives to get away from the physical world through the pursuit of enjoyment, pleasure, and identification with others. Enjoyment of the sensory organs is the impelling force of his life so long as he vibrates here. This is the plane of wine, women, and song. Sexuality becomes a primary means of self-expression—which can be a tremendous drain on the vital energies.

The player dwells in the worlds of feeling, emotion, idea, and meaning and uses them as the basis of his fantasies. Thus the second chakra is the starting point of all the creative arts. Fantasy is the power behind creativity.

The astral plane is the dimension of psychic space midway between heaven and earth. The player has dwelt on the lower levels, and his imagination brings the possibility of heaven within reach. The danger is that he may let himself be carried away by his fantasies, which drain his energy and leave him exhausted.

15
Plane of fantasy
(naga-loka)

Naga-loka was supposed to be the underworld. As there are seven *lokas* above, so are there seven below. *Lokas* below are situated under water. The ruler of each underworld is a different kind of being. One of these seven is Patal. The rulers of one region are serpents *(nagas)*. In mythology these *nagas* are supposed to be semidivine beings with a human face and the tail of a dragon. *Nagas* also exist as a sect of initiate hermits who are masters of great wisdom: nothing is hidden or could be hidden from them. Thus *naga-loka* is the plane of fantasy. It is not above the physical plane but below—submerged under water in accordance with the nature of fantasy.

The player who lands here enters fully into the realm of the fantastic.

Here his imagination soars wholly beyond the physical plane and into the infinite potentialities of human existence. He sees no limits on his nature. There is nothing he cannot do. He pours his energies into exploring his fantasies; emerging with works of art and new ideas and inventions. He explores the world his senses present to him, seeking ever more stimulation for his imagination. He uses his sensory input to create new combinations never before experienced. Here is the plane of speculation, of "What if?" No restraints are placed on the bounds of the imagination. Nothing is too fantastic or bizarre to be considered.

In entertainment the player became aware of possibilities. On the plane of fantasy he is immersed in them. Many of the finest works of art have come from this surrender to the unrestrained imagination. But if the imagination is allowed to soar too high and too long, the player loses contact with the reality of his everyday life—and the snake of jealousy lurks just ahead, to catch him if he becomes too caught up in the fantastic to see what lies before him.

In Sanskrit *naga* means snake. Thus the plane of fantasy is also the snake plane. The snake is synonymous with energy. The *kundalini,* which the yogi seeks to raise through his efforts, is often called the serpent power. The devil often appears in the guise of a snake. The snake is the embodiment of movement and the animal that best represents the nature of the player vibrating in the second chakra. It implies flexibility and the protean ability to change form. As the snake seeks shelter in the hollows of the earth, so does the player who lands in the second chakra.

16

Jealousy

(dwesh)

When the player allows his fantasies to carry him away, the resulting loss of energy can bring him to the square of jealousy—the basic second-chakra problem. Jealousy is a condition of mental imbalance resulting from suspicion and the fear of rivalry and unfaithfulness. It is a form of insanity, which troubles the mind of the self-intoxicated player. His ability to fantasize allows him to swell his ego out of all proportion. He loses the ability to distinguish between what is possible and what is. His confusion stems from his overindulgence in the fantastic.

He begins to suspect others when they fail to conform to his own self-image. In love he is jealous and fearful of rivals. His self-doubts grow, and soon his energy is drawn back to the first chakra, where he becomes caught up in greed. Jealousy nurtured his lack of self-confidence, which bore fruit as insecurity, the basic first-chakra character trait. His lack of self-confidence also leads to self-hatred, which is then projected outward as the hatred of others.

To regain his sense of self-confidence he must reexperience the first chakra, where he can lose his insecurity and again raise his vibrations.

17

Mercy
(daya)

Mercy is a divine attribute present in the player, holding such power that it moves him directly from the second chakra to the eighth, and the Absolute plane. Mercy is a surrender to compassion of such potency that the ego is swept aside in an outrush of feeling so intense that the eyes fill with tears of joy and the heart pulses in exultation and cosmic love. For the moment he is at one with the Divine.

Mercy is the most positive face of the second-chakra ability to imagine possibilities. The state of mercy is created when compassion is extended to one through whom the player's self-identification was injured. Instead of striking back, taking an "I for an I," the player turns the other cheek.

The ability to imagine gives the player insight into the motivations of others. The player sees that it was he himself who allowed the hurt, that the other was not responsible. He knows that both he and the other are players in a cosmic game far beyond their present level of comprehension. He sees that he too could have caused the injury to another. He recognizes that there are higher levels of vibration, and that only one who attains the insights gained in vibrating on those planes can judge another. He extends this, the essence of compassion, to the other player in the form of forgiveness. This very realization frees his consciousness from self-identification, and he soars up to the Absolute plane.

In Sanskrit there is a saying: *daya* (mercy) is the foundation-stone of dharma (righteousness). Without mercy a truly religious nature is not possible. Mercy, kindness, forbearance, temperance—all in time enrich the good in man and help him in the refining of his emotions, the formation of his character, and his ethical development. The barrier of personality is swept away, and his mind becomes a reflection of the Divine. Mercy is a surrender. However, an act of mercy cannot eliminate all past karmas, so the player must roll until the snake of *tamoguna* bites him. Then he is swallowed and taken back to earth to fulfill his mission.

18

Plane of joy
(harsha-loka)

Here at the end of the second row, the second plane, the second chakra, comes a feeling of deep satisfaction. The player knows he has moved away from envy, nullity, and jealousy. He is moving away from the realm of fantasy to encounter the real world, the stage of karma yoga. He does not know how soon he will reach his goal, Cosmic Consciousness, but he knows that the levels of being can be transcended, that the energy can be raised. The feeling of anticipation for his encounter with the world quickens him, and he begins to feel deeply on every level of being. There is a challenge ahead of him, but there is also the abiding satisfaction that comes with completion. One phase has ended; another is about to begin.

It is at this moment of transcendence that the spirit of joy pervades his being.

He has passed the first chakra; there is no fear, no insecurity. He has completed the second chakra; he has risen above sensual desires. What lies ahead is the joyous task of karma yoga. He feels on top of himself and the world. He is fired by the spirit of the quest. The sense of time disappears. Joy is always eternal, however brief its duration. The awareness of space passes away. Joy knows no limits. But the joy cannot last forever. Soon the forces of karma begin to work, and the task of moving through the third level begins.

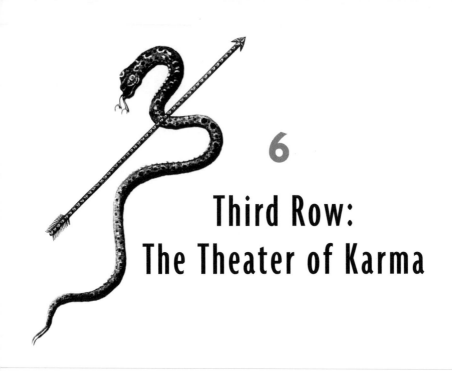

6

Third Row:
The Theater of Karma

19
Plane of action
(karma-loka)

This, the plane of action, begins the third row of the game and the exploration of the third chakra. The only desire that remains true for all times and places is the desire for fulfillment. All other desires are manifestations of that one desire: the desire for completion, for self-realization. So on whatever level the player vibrates, on that level does he seek fulfillment.

In the first and second chakras the desire was manifested as the pursuit of money and sex. In the third chakra the dominant concern becomes identification of the ego and achievement of power. First-chakra people work neither for themselves nor on themselves. They are usually employed in aiding the fulfillment of some third-chakra person. In the second chakra, desire flows in the direction of the senses, and the exploration of the sensual realm consumes the energy. It is in the third chakra that the player becomes conscious of the social and political influences on the development of his personality. Thus the player becomes self-conscious. Egotism becomes the impetus of action, as the ego seeks to extend its influence in ever-broadening circles. In this fashion *karma-loka* makes one face reality from a more realistic perspective. Second-chakra fantasies fall before the practicalities of the world. It is a moment of sobriety. At this point one becomes aware of the law of karma.

Each thing is in a constant state of interaction with all other things. On the level of energy, karma determines the frequency of vibration, which on the gross level is manifested as the player's behavior patterns. Karma is the cause of the cycle of birth and rebirth. And karma alone can win for the player liberation from the cycle, creating both bondage and liberation.

Basically, the player has karmic responsibility for his self. This self can be divided into manifested and unmanifested, body and being. So there are karmas toward the body and karmas toward consciousness. Body is world: body contains all the elements of gross manifestation. So karmas toward the body are karmas toward the whole world. Consciousness is the essence of the world; so karmas toward consciousness also cover the whole world.

20
Charity
(daan)

Those karmas that raise the vibrational level are known as virtues; those that lower it are vices. Charity is a human virtue that exists on the third-chakra level. It lifts the player above the problems of the third chakra and transports him to the fourth level of the game, the plane of balance.

As a virtue, charity is a manifestation of the Divinity, which is the essence of consciousness. When the player lands on this square,

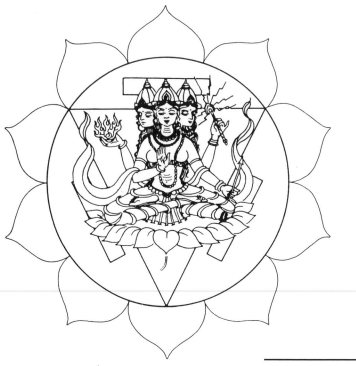

The theater of karma

he identifies with the Divinity—present in all—and performs acts of charity without desiring any personal benefit from his karma.

A feeling of elation is experienced during the performance of the act of charity. This is the raising of energy from a lower level to a higher one. That is why all human religions have stressed the significance of charity and included charitable acts in their rituals. The reality of need and the desire to share are the two factors at work at the base of the game. Charity satisfies the developing ego and breaks the bondage of third chakra.

Charity is one of the most important pillars of the plane of karma. It is the motivating force behind man's highest institutionalized activities—the mergence of compassion with the third-chakra penchant for organization.

21

Atonement

(saman paap)

When the player has risen above the press of material and sensual desires, he gains the awareness that in the course of gratifying his lower needs he has caused harm to others. He has acted blindly in his search for fulfillment, without awareness of the consequences of his actions. When he lands on the plane of atonement he sees that by the use of wrong actions and wrong means he has created wrong vibrations within himself, which prevent the attainment of inner peace.

In search of that inner peace he lands in atonement to make up for the wrongs he has done, to make up for errors in conduct, to atone for his follies. It is a time of great emotional turmoil. There is a keen and pressing desire to rectify the negative karmas, the vices he has entertained.

Atonement is also the square for second-chakra personalities who have landed in the third chakra and feel guilty for their inability to adjust to vibrating at a higher level. In both cases, atonement produces positive results and helps in the upward flow of energy. The player atones by following the law of dharma, which is the true nature of everything. Atonement puts one in tune with dharma—which is the next square of the game.

22

Plane of dharma

(dharma-loka)

Dharma is whatever is right. Dharma is an ever-evolving, ever-flowing principle. Dharma is an atemporal, aspatial force working in human existence. Dharma is constant, but its form varies from situation to situation. It lives in the depths of reality. The player who finds the stream of dharma dwells in reality and becomes at one with it (at-one-ment follows atonement).

Conscious action is dharma—conscious action in accord with the reality of the moment. Learning to act consciously is learning to act in accord with the principles of the cosmos. So dharma is that action which accords with cosmic knowledge.

There are ten signposts of dharma, all of which must be present if the action is to accord with the law of dharma: firmness, forgiveness, self-command, restraint (nonstealing), cleanliness (purity), control of the sensory and work organs, intellect, right knowledge, truth, and absence of anger.

Whatever you feel is genuinely good for yourself is good for others. There is no dharma like doing good for others. There is no *adharma,* vice, worse than causing harm to another. Dharma can best be understood when related to conduct. Yet it is far more than a code of conduct, of morality and ethics. These are attributes of dharma but not all of dharma. Ethics is a reflection of dharma, not dharma itself.

The dharma of fire is to burn. The dharma of water is to quench. It is the dharma of water to create taste, as it is the dharma of fire to create color and form. The innate, essential nature of a thing is its dharma. And there is no escape from dharma. The moment there is a deviation the energy flows downward, drawing the player down with it. The arrows on this board are dharmas, virtues; the snakes *adharmas,* vices.

Though dharma exists always, beyond form, it assumes a special form for each player. It is the dharma of the player who lives in a cold climate to wear warm clothing. It is the dharma of the hungry man to take nourishment. It is the dharma of the student to meditate and partake of *sadhana,* spiritual discipline. It is the dharma of the child to play freely, without care for the world of the spirit. It is the dharma of the elderly to dwell in the realm of spirit. Dharma is the truth that holds all existence in proper relationship.

Dharma is the scaffolding on which is constructed the edifice of the self. As long as the building is not complete, the scaffolding holds the structure erect. The minute the building becomes self-supporting the scaffolding is removed and used for other unstable, evolving new buildings.

23
Celestial plane
(swarga-loka)

Swarga-loka, the heaven world, is the third *loka* of the seven planes of existence. These three—*bhu-loka, bhuvar-loka,* and *swarga-loka*—belong to a category of planes that perish at the end of a day of creation—a day of the Creator, Brahma—and are reborn with the dawn of the succeeding day. On *bhu-loka,* the physical plane, all exists on a physical level; on *bhuvar-loka,* the astral plane, the desires are at work; and on *swarga-loka,* the celestial plane, work is carried out at the level of thoughts. On this plane the fire element is the ruling power, and all that exists on this level of existence is made up of particles of fire—luminous, lustrous particles of light—and that is why the beings in *swarga-loka* are self luminous. Shining angels and gods are mentioned everywhere in all mythologies.

In the first chakra the player longed for security and sought possessions that would protect and nurture him. In the second chakra he explored the world of the senses and strove for sensual gratification. On reaching the level of the third chakra he begins to see beyond the material and sensual realms and to fathom the nature of his ego, his personal identity. So here the concern is that of providing immortality for his identity-construct.

Once this desire for ego-immortality springs into his heart, the celestial laws attract his attention as he tries to fashion for himself a heaven from his own desires. The heaven he conceives is a plane full of all that his self requires for pleasure, joy, and happiness. He realistically sees the world as full of pain and suffering, rises and falls. He craves a pleasure that is infinite, without cessation or variation. This is the space known as heaven, nurtured by the religions of all peoples. Even Marx, that atheistic third-chakra philosopher, could not do without a heaven. He called his ultimate goal the classless society.

Heaven is a manifestation of third-chakra desire. If we detach ourselves from value judgments we can see it as a genuinely higher plane, one attained from the second chakra by purification. Heaven is the lure used to sway errant first- and second-chakra sheep back into the spiritual fold, and it has been used by saints and prophets of all religions to raise the spiritual level of the masses.

In the Hindu tradition heaven is the domain of Indra. He is the one who has mastered his *indryas*, the five organs of perception and the five organs of action. One who masters these organs becomes lord of Heaven and dwells in this space. Heaven is the dwelling place of saints, *bhaktas* (spiritual devotees), high karma-yogis, and the celestial dancers and musicians (see square 11).

To one who has mastered his organs of perception and action, everything exists as it does on the physical plane but in harmonious and divine form. There are no lower desires, no violence, no attachment, no greed, no jealousy, no avarice, no anger, no sensuality, no nullity. There exist instead purification, recreation, mercy, joy, and an infinite life to enjoy. Heaven is the edifice constructed with the scaffolding of dharma.

24

Bad company
(ku-sang-loka)

In the search for ego identification that characterizes third-chakra activities, the player seeks out groups to support him in his quest. He is aware that alone he lacks the strength to fulfill his desire, and he seeks others on a similar path to form a mutually supporting group.

If he is vibrating wrongly, he may find himself in a group that does not act in accord with dharma. Then he finds himself in bad company, a snake that bites him and takes him down to the first chakra and conceit.

In bad company his wrong character traits are either ignored or extolled. The power generated by group activities may cause his ego to swell and his selfishness to grow. He deceives himself into thinking his actions are in accord with dharma. The further he deviates from the path, the greater his conceit grows. He soon finds himself back in the first chakra and must seek purification or entertainment.

In bad company, personal problems are seen as caused by others. The terrorist, the political conspirator who resorts to any means to attain his aim, is the extreme example. He is deluded by those in his circle into thinking that assassination is correct. He feels that by killing another he can fulfill the desire within himself. He sees his own aims as the right aims for everyone. This deviation from dharma, this gross abuse of personal power, is a characteristic third-chakra problem. This abuse draws his energy down.

Bad company is *adharma*. Only by acting in accord with dharma can the player extricate himself from this trap.

25

Good company
(su-sang-loka)

The player who begins to follow the path of dharma in the third chakra soon begins to find himself in the company of others who are seeking to realize that which is best in themselves. Within this group, the player finds his energies raised by the affirmation that comes from knowing others are seeking the same goal. His third-chakra quest, extending his ego, takes a new turn. This positive association, this good company, is *su-sang*.

For the one who seeks to realize spiritual values within himself, *su-sang* usually takes the form of an organic fellowship formed around the person and teachings of a fourth- or fifth-chakra person. Bad company usually revolves around a charismatic third-chakra leader. The player and those in his group cooperate to emulate their teacher, to incorporate what the teacher gives into their own identities.

In good company vices are not extolled. The players, with the aid of the master, serve as mirrors for each other so that both good and bad tendencies can be observed and acted upon. While conceit is the outcome of bad company, compassion develops from good company.

Good company is essential for the player. It provides him with the opportunity to grow away from old identifications in an atmosphere of trust and compassion. Vestiges of first- and second-chakra problems gradually disappear as he learns to confront and work with all aspects of his self.

Good company is the positive side of the third-chakra drive for affiliation and identification. There are no more traps to bar his way to the fourth level of the game, the plane of cosmic mind and balance.

26
Sorrow
(dukh)

Sorrow is the term used to describe the alteration in body chemistry created by a loss. This loss of energy (or pressure) creates a state of depression in the organism. Sorrow and joy represent two ends of the emotional continuum. Joy is a state of expansion, extroversion, and elevated vibrations; sorrow is a state of contraction, introversion, and depressed vibrations. In both, the sense of time vanishes, and the moment seems eternal.

In sorrow the breathing is constricted and repressed. The blood is drawn inward to the vital organs. The complexion is one of pallor. In joy the breathing is unrestrained and fluid. The heart opens and blood courses throughout the body. The complexion is glowing, vibrant, vital.

Sorrow is a blanket, which wraps the player in its folds and blinds his vision. He cannot see anything outside the blanket. No ray of hope and no light can penetrate. The more the player fights to extricate himself, the deeper he finds himself entangled. He feels himself weak, helpless. He is torn between his intellect, which tells him there is a way out, and his feelings, which proclaim the state eternal.

All that is required of him is to stand up and throw off the blanket once and for all. There is clear sky outside; but within the heavy woolly karmic blanket there exists only confusion and the complexes created by fantasy. Like a child afraid of the dark, cowering under his blanket, he imagines dark terrors lurking just outside, ready to consume him if he but shows himself.

Sorrow can be a temporary state, as in the sorrow created by the seemingly senseless murder of a child, the innocents slaughtered in war. Or it can become the way of being, a permanent imbalance in body chemistry created through the mechanism of suppression.

When suppression is at work, the player knows there is an aspect of himself he does not choose to confront. Confronting it means loss of identity, acceptance of the unacceptable. Yet suppression creates pain. The blocked energy must express itself, and pain becomes the medium. Here sorrow is the dragon that swallows its own tail. Expression of the inexpressible would create pain and loss of identity. Nonexpression also brings pain, confusion, and the loss of identity.

In *sadhana,* following a spiritual discipline, sorrow can be a manifestation of the awareness of separation between devotee and deity. The third chakra is the plane of identification. The aspirant seeks to identify with his deity. Repeated failure brings him to sorrow. The player feels an awareness of the Divine, and craves nothing more than the realization of that Divinity within himself. Yet the separation seems an impassable chasm. He sees the first- and second-chakra problems that repeatedly trap his energy. He senses the Divine yet feels himself unworthy, unable to know it.

There is a way out, and selfless service, the next square, offers hope.

27
Selfless service
(parmarth)

Charity is an action, performed frequently or infrequently. Selfless service is an attitude, a mode of being. *Parmarth* is living without the self yet harmoniously with the world, while doing a right job and retaining consciousness of the moment.

Parm means supreme. *Arth* is meaning, the purpose for which an action is performed. That which is done for the supreme is *parmarth*. Supreme may mean God, or it may mean a cause for which the player chooses to dedicate his existence. It is a giving up of self for a higher cause.

When a player understands his role in the drama and knows that the individual self is but a vehicle for realization of the Supreme, all that he does ceases to concern him. He only does his duty and acts out his role in the play. He does not know what the final outcome of his actions will be. When he does his duty without thought of right or reward he becomes selfless. And then all his acts are *parmarth*.

Living in *parmarth* is possible only when the player realizes that rights follow duty and that rewards are the fruits of action. Duty and honor (rewards) are byproducts of the game, not the final goal. As long as the player exists within a body with five organs of action, karmas are inevitable. The player's choice is whether to become concerned about rewards and punishment, honor and humiliation, or to devote his life to understanding the nature of the game and living unconcerned with whatever happens, continuing to perform his duty.

A reward is in nobody's hand. Countless factors affect the outcome of every momentary situation. Whatever happens is whatever was possible at that time. If the player has no hopes and desires, every moment becomes an achievement. When he gets away from the false concepts of profit and loss, he enters on to the plane of selfless service.

Selfless service is an arrow that lifts the player to the human plane. Performing his duty in a right manner, giving up the self to what has to be done, brings about the loss of identification that is the greatest problem in the third chakra. The individual ceases to exist as a separate entity and becomes part of a larger whole.

Examples of this third-chakra selfless service can be found in organizations—one of the primary forms of expression on the celestial plane. Charitable institutions, grant foundations, and professional volunteer service groups all constitute forms of selfless service. Selfless service is exemplified in the lives of Albert Schweitzer, Martin Luther King Jr., and Nathan Hale ("I regret that I have but one life to give for my country").

Selfless service is the last plane through which the player must pass in the third row of the game, the third chakra. From here he moves on to the plane of balance, the plane of faith and devotion.

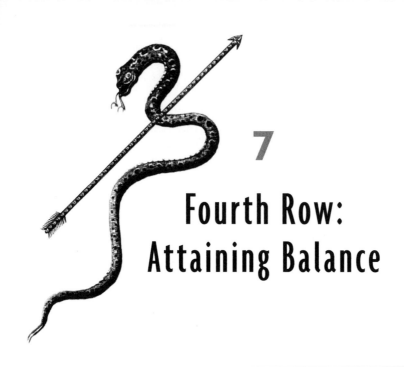

7

Fourth Row: Attaining Balance

28
Apt religion
(sudharma)

Sudharma, apt religion, means adoption of the course of action best suited to the player's own self. *Sudharma* is living in harmony with the laws of the game. It is the course of action that allows the player to throw his die without care of where he lands.

Sudharma literally means one's own dharma. What is one's dharma? What is one supposed to do? If dharma is a code of conduct, then it should be common to everyone. Then nobody would have to do any thinking. Everyone would adopt the same mode of living. But people are people, not machines. They have individual differences, and those differences are the products of numerous factors. Not everyone is born at the same time or of the same parents. Parentage, environment, atmosphere, latitude and longitude, and geographical, anthropological and sociological conditions differ from individual to individual. Everyone is born with a set of qualifications and disqualifications.

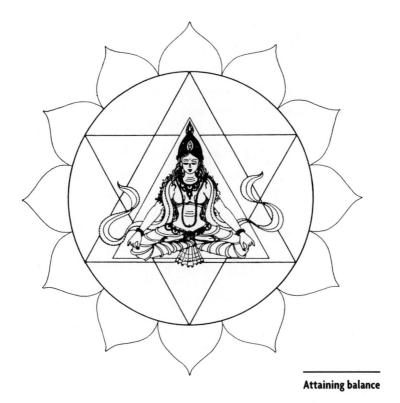

Attaining balance

Ideal is not real. No one can completely submerge himself in the law of dharma prescribed by a particular religion or individual. Everybody has to understand his role in the game. He has to follow his own path to liberation. The rise and fall in each individual life determines the course of play.

Sudharma means to keep up the spirit that one is ever evolving while never adopting unfair means in the course of action. *Sudharma* is to believe in liberation, in merging with Cosmic Consciousness. *Sudharma* is nonattachment to the rise and fall of maya.

If the player is a musician he will find his *sudharma* in music. A painter will find his through his own art. There are seven psychic centers in which the player vibrates. Wherever he feels comfortable, there he should try to evolve his energies into new patterns. This is the only *sudharma*. All religious codes of conduct are but external aids in the task of understanding one's true nature, one's *sudharma*. Once the player begins to understand his *sudharma*, religion becomes internal, a way of life. Rituals lose their import. Life itself becomes an act of worship. The player is ready to move on to the plane of austerity.

Until the player lands in the fourth chakra, dharma is a meaningless term. He has to identify with a group or ideology in the third chakra. In the second he identifies with his senses; in the first with his ability to ensure bodily survival.

In the third chakra he understands karma, charity, the dharma aspect called ethics, good and bad company, atonement, the sorrows of life, and selfless service. But an understanding of his own role in the game starts only when he lands in the fourth chakra, in *sudharma*. *Sudharma* leads him to the plane of austerity and to hard penance and work on himself. Following the path of *sudharma* leads him directly to the sixth row of the game, the sixth chakra.

29
Irreligiosity
(adharma)

The player who lands in *sudharma* discovers his true role in the game and acts out his part without regard to the outcome of his actions. He knows that as long as he listens to the voice of his own inner nature he need fear nothing.

Faith in accordance with the laws of nature is *sudharma*. Blind faith, which disregards the cosmic principles, leads to *adharma*. *Adharmas* are those actions which are contrary to the individual's dharma. *Adharmas* lead him away from his true course and back into first chakra delusion, which is the essence of blind faith.

Adharma is working contrary to the laws of existence. At sunrise everything on the planet changes. Winds, atmospheric pressures, and temperatures change. The tempo of life increases. Sleeping at this time is acting contrary to the laws of the planet. Thus it is *adharma*. Looting the earth for natural resources, which are then employed without concern for their negative effects on the environment and the future needs of the planet, is *adharma* against the earth. Similarly, there are *adharmas* related to one's own physiology. To hold tension and not release it is *adharma*. But to release it by adopting unfair means is greater *adharma*.

Adharma does not exist by itself. It is a negation of the law of dharma, an action contrary to the true inner nature. Denying one's own self is *adharma*. Self-rejection and self-praise are both *adharmas*. To understand one's position in the game is *sudharma*. All else is *adharma*.

Adharma is best understood as an imbalance in the *gunas*, the three primary cosmic forces responsible for all manifestation. When either *sattva* (conscious energy), *tamas* (inertia), or *rajas* (motion) predominates, *adharma* takes birth. Self-destruction is the greatest *adharma*. It is a snake that takes one back to delusion, back to the start of the game.

The danger of getting caught by *adharma* is greatest in the fourth chakra, the fourth row of the game. In the first three chakras energy was devoted to the physical, celestial, and astral planes. Now, in the fourth chakra, the player attains a degree of balance and begins to understand the importance of apt religion. While he seeks his own role in the game it is possible that he might ignore the existing dharmas and attempt to start his own way, ignoring planetary laws and the laws of existence. Here faith is the key.

Faith is the essence of fourth chakra: faith, devotion, *bhakti*. This faith can lead the player—if he acts in harmony with his true nature, *sudharma*—to the plane of austerity. But if it is not in tune with his innermost vibrations, it can draw him back to delusion. This is *adharma*. Acting on faith alone is liable to create irreligiosity. Faith alone, without a grounding in the laws of existence, is blind faith. And blind faith is the most frequent cause of energy loss in this plane. Faith in accordance with the laws of existence is *sudharma,* but faith alone is *adharma.*

30
Good tendencies
(uttam gati)

Uttam is good; *gati* is movement. Good tendencies flow spontaneously when the player moves in harmony with the laws of the macrocosm. When the player vibrates in the lower chakras, good tendencies do not develop. They are found here in the heart chakra, the fourth row of the game. Only when the player reaches a degree of balance within himself can good tendencies arise spontaneously. This balance enables the player to tune his own vibratory rate with that of the cosmos. Good tendencies are movements in the direction of increasingly finer tuning.

In the fourth chakra, heart and breath play a significant role. By landing in good tendencies the player attains control over his own breath pattern and simultaneously his heart rate. Good tendencies therefore help in stabilizing the development of the fourth chakra, and breath is directly related to good tendencies.

Any change in direction (or tendency) is registered by the *prana,* the life-force, psychic energy, or *élan vital.* On a gross level this change is experienced as a change in respiration. Each wrong breath pattern is an injury to the organism. Thus, when the player spoils his breathing cycle he simultaneously creates bad vibratory frequencies within himself. Good tendencies are a device to help the player keep vibrating correctly. They can be identified by observing one's own breath pattern.

The best tendencies are those that link the player ever more closely to the rhythm cycles of the planet and the cosmos. Begin by observing changes in the self at sunrise and sunset. Arise before dawn, in time to shower and change into clean clothes for sunrise meditation. Other good tendencies include the elimination of meat and eggs from the diet, the practice of *hatha yoga asanas* (postures and exercises), the regulation of breathing (see the *lokas* of *prana, apana,* and *uyana*), fasting, conscientious study of spiritual writings, and all the virtues contained in the game of Leela, the yoga of snakes and arrows.

The practice of good tendencies helps the player stabilize his existence so that it flows rhythmically in positive directions and away from the energy-depleting distractions of the lower chakras.

31
Plane of sanctity
(yaksha-loka)

The player who lands on the plane of sanctity experiences divine grace through the understanding and knowledge of cosmic principles. Sanctity is a direct result of good tendencies. It is the fourth-chakra feeling of oneness with the presence of Divinity, and the ability to perceive the divine grace in all existence. This oneness passes beyond mere intellectual understanding and becomes an actual part of daily life.

Yakshas were celestial beings who dwelt in heaven. According to Hindu cosmology, creation is divided into seven classes of being: *devas, yakshas* (or *kinnaras*), *gandharvas, manushyas, asuras* (or *rakshas*), *bhootas,* and *pishachas. Pishachas* represent the lowest type of consciousness, the essence of which is meanness and violence. Next are the *bhootas,* or ghosts. These are disincarnate beings unable to detach from the plane of earthly existence, living in the past. Then come the *asuras,* beings who do not believe in a code of ethical conduct and who live in search of sensual gratification—wine, women, and song. Then come the *manushyas,* who believe in the law of karma and responsibility for the consequences of their actions. *Manushyas* are aware of the future and of the nature of liberation. This is the plane of human existence. Then come the *gandharvas,* who are consciousness devoted to the service of the gods and living in harmony with the divine music. *Gandharvas* dedicate their existence to elevating people through sound and music. Then comes the class of *yakshas,* a kind of consciousness grounded in the knowledge and understanding of cosmic principles and direct experience of the divine grace. Lastly are the *devas,* the pure energy forms of the gods themselves.

When the player lands in *yaksha-loka,* questions about the nature of divine existence draw his attention. He seeks to find the links between the divine and his daily life. Only on reaching the fourth chakra is the Divinity reached on an experiential level. Before then, it has been but an abstract concept. This curiosity about the Divine and its presence in all existence, this desire to confront reality, becomes the essence of the player.

32
Plane of balance
(maha- or *mahar-loka)*

Mahar-loka is the fourth *loka* of the seven levels of existence. This *loka* is regarded as perishing at the Night of Brahma, the Creator. The first three *lokas* are those in which the *jiva* (individual consciousness) lives during the course of its evolution and is subject to the wheel of births and deaths. In this fourth *loka* the fire element is again predominant, but now it is not as elegant as in *swarga-loka,* where the bodies of its dwellers are luminous and flashing. Here the player is above the physical, desire, and thought levels. Individual consciousness is colored by desires *(kama)* and thoughts, but now that the player has reached the state of being desireless and thoughtless, he has transcended the third level and reached the fourth, the permanent invisible world. Those who dwell here are not absolutely free from transmigration, but they will not be reborn in this cycle of creation because they exist in balance.

Three centers above and three below make this, the plane of the heart chakra, the balancing point of the spine of the game. From here, energy flows downward to the first three centers and upward to the higher three planes of being. Here is the center where the male and female energies are balanced. The player who vibrates in the fourth chakra speaks from the heart.

He reaches *maha-loka* through the arrow of charity, or by passing through good tendencies and the plane of sanctity. Here the desires of the lower chakras are stilled, and energy is no longer exhausted in the pursuit of lower aims. From the heart begins the upward flow of energy.

Here also the player transcends the intellectual understanding of Divinity that characterizes the third chakra and moves into a direct experience of the Divine within himself. Because of this sense of unity with the Absolute, it has also been called the plane of Cosmic Mind.

The heart center has long been recognized as the most important seat of feeling in the body. The heart is the dwelling-place of the emotional self. Yoga physiology attributes this fact to the location of the ductless thymus gland in the heart region. This gland is responsible for the flow of electrical energy in the body—and the nature of sense perception is fundamentally electrical. Each change in emotional tone is registered by the heart, and the pattern in which the heart beats determines body chemistry. Each change in body chemistry is understood by the mind as a certain type of feeling or emotion.

Thus the heart is more than a machine to pump pure blood into the body and convey waste-charged blood back to the lungs. It is also a center of feeling, a psychic center. The Sufi tradition also stresses the importance of opening the heart chakra through love, or *mohabbat*. From here poetry begins, the transformation of the personal into the impersonal. Poetry is full of heart—its vibrations, its different feelings. This center is also the source of all transpersonal psychic phenomena.

By whatever path he lands here, the player now feels relaxed. His hands automatically start making the gestures *(mudras)* that help balance the flow of energy through his organism. His heart becomes filled with the devotional spirit, *bhakti*. He is able to begin to identify himself with the rest of creation, bringing on a sense of cosmic unity. Tender feelings and a sense of aesthetics become manifested in his behavior. The player's voice becomes softer and gentler as he starts to speak from the heart. His voice penetrates the hearts of others, and thus without any exertion of power he attracts to himself a group of admirers striving to reach the same vibrational patterns.

The symbol of the plane of balance is a six-pointed star composed of two equilateral triangles, one pointing upward and the other pointing down. The upward-pointing triangle of this Star of David (as it has become known in the West) signifies male energy; the downward, female. This implies the balance between the two energies attained by the player who vibrates here.

Hindu cosmology enumerates fourteen major planes, *lokas,* seven of which are regions rising above the earth. They are the planes of the seven chakras that constitute the spine of this game—as well as the player's own physical spine. First is *bhu-loka,* the physical plane. Second is *bhuvar-loka,* the astral plane. Third is *swarga-loka,* the celestial plane. Fourth is *maha-loka,* the plane of balance. *Jana-loka,* the human plane, is fifth, followed by *tapa-loka,* the plane of austerity, and *satya-loka,* the plane of reality. The lower regions descending from the earth are *atal-loka, vital-loka, sutal-loka, rasatal-loka, talatal-loka, mahatal-loka,* and *patal-loka.*

In everyday Hindu worship *(sandhya)* the supplicant recites a mantra (chant), which enumerates each of the seven major *lokas.* As he voices the name of each plane he touches the part of the body with which it is associated. He chants *Om bhu* as with the moistened tip of the right ring-finger he touches the midpoint between anus and genitals, the seat of the *kundalini.* Then he chants *Om bhuvah* as he touches the root of the genitals, the seat of the second psychic center. The chant *Om swah* accompanies the touching of the navel. He intones *Om maha* as he touches his heart, *Om janah* for the base of the throat, and *Om tapah* for the third eye, the midpoint between the eyes and slightly above the eyebrows. Last is *Om satyam,* the top of the head.

33

Plane of fragrance
(gandha-loka)

Gandha means smell, and the sense of smell is linked with the earth and the physical plane. Once the player reaches the fourth level, however, the nature of the sense is transmuted and becomes the symbol of the Divine, carrying a strong emotional impact. In the course of *sudharma* the devotee offers scents to the deity, in the form of either flowers or incense. Thus the fourth chakra contains the plane of fragrance, *gandha-loka*.

In the first chakra, odors like petroleum, paraffin, and alcohol attract the player. In the second chakra he is stimulated by strong-smelling synthetic preparations. In the third chakra these same artificial scents predominate, but they are now far more costly. When he reaches the plane of balance he realizes the futility of the inorganic, and avoids pungent, artificial odors.

Here in *gandha-loka* he experiences divine fragrances in his meditation. The evolution of energy effects a change in body chemistry, and his organism ceases to produce bad odors, exuding instead a fragrance not unlike that of lotus flowers or sandalwood.

As a measure of understanding, the *sadhak* (devotee) is asked to stop the use of artificial scents on his body so that he comes to know his own odors. When his body stops smelling bad, and when his stool, sweat, and breath produce no bad odors, he knows his energy has transcended the third chakra and entered into the plane of fragrance.

Now there are only divine odors. Once and for all, the player has eliminated bad odors from his system.

34

Plane of taste
(rasa-loka)

While in the lower chakras the sense of taste was predominantly a mode of sensory perception, in the fourth chakra it becomes purified—taste in the aesthetic sense. One who lands in this plane is able to penetrate into the world of ideas and meanings. This penetration gives the player direct experiential knowledge of the essence of emotions and sentiments.

Rasa is love, pleasure, grace, enjoyment, sentiment, taste, emotions, beauty, passion, spirit. It is the poetic sentiment, the essence of poetry. *Rasa* is water in its purest form, the force that binds all creation together.

Up to the third chakra, taste—in all its shades of meaning—is devoted to lower-level activities. In the first chakra the sense of taste is totally dominated by the desire to make money. Power foods (meat especially) and prepared foods (convenience products) are the basis of the player's diet. He uses a great deal of salt and spice. By the second chakra the energies are diverted toward sensuality, especially sex. Here foods that increase sexual stamina, such as eggs, ginseng, and fish, are his concern. In the third chakra he indulges taste for its own sake, consuming foods for different flavors and textures. But in the fourth chakra, the heart plane, the sense of taste becomes purified. He leaves salt and sweet tastes to understand the real essence of the food he consumes.

Once the player lands on the plane of taste, his taste improves in all dimensions. His tastes in food, music, and conversation are pleasing to all, regardless of their vibrational level. He becomes a master of good taste, appreciated by all. Thus he draws to himself a group of admirers who seek to vibrate in the same frequencies.

35
Purgatory
(narka-loka)

Until the player reaches the level of the heart chakra he lacks understanding of *sudharma,* apt religion. Without *sudharma,* freedom of action is impossible. As the player attains freedom of action he becomes responsible for the fruits of his actions. *Narka-loka* is the place where he bears those consequences.

In Hindu cosmology *narka* is a plane situated midway between earth and heaven. There are seven layers of *narka-loka* that the player must pass through before attaining heaven. His karmas are the vehicle, leading him up to the level where they vibrate. After passing through these *narkas,* if the player has performed good karmas he is ready to pass into heaven.

The lord of *narka* is Yama, known as *Dharmaraj*—the lord of death. Violence leads the player to purgatory and to the most painful vibrational levels. Each action bears fruit. This is the law of karma, and it cannot be avoided as long as the player maintains a physical existence. When the player lands in *narka-loka* through bad karmas he is bound to this plane by karmic ties. This is not punishment but rather purification. *Dharmaraj,* the lord of *narka,* is not personally interested in the suffering of any player. He is not a sadistic devil. Rather, his job is to set wrong frequencies right so that future evolution of the spirit can take place.

Narka is also the heart chakra itself. Attachment to feelings is *narka.* The feeling of attachment is *narka. Narka* is negative vibration. Those who vibrate negatively create a *narka* in their home, family, neighborhood, town, country, and world, according to their capacity. The player who lands in *narka-loka* without fourth chakra understanding sees it as failure, not as a record of negative karma. Only in the fourth chakra does the understanding of negative karmas on the experiential level come. The *narka-loka* is seen not as the result of personal ego failure but as the sign of an imperfection of action and the need to improve. In the fourth chakra comes recognition without valuation.

36
Clarity of consciousness
(swatch)

Clarity of consciousness is the light that illuminates the player on his passage out of the fourth row of the game and on to the fifth, the plane where man becomes Man. *Swatch* in Sanskrit means clear, pure, transparent. This transparency results from the purification of the opacities of bad karmas the player undergoes in purgatory.

Transparency offers no resistance to the passage of light. When doubts are clarified, the fog of blind intellect is dissolved to be replaced by the clear, strong light of inner feelings. The intellectual understanding, which dominates the consciousness up to the third chakra, does so no more. Reason here is considered an ailment, a disease of consciousness. For when consciousness identifies itself with understanding, at that time it suffers from the disease of reason, the chains of the intellect. By devotion and right faith the disease is overcome, and the player enters into the realm of Being.

When the player lands here he becomes *swatch*—clear, pure, transparent. The doubts that assailed him took him to purgatory and irreligiosity. But from those experiences he gained an understanding of the nature of *sudharma*. He has developed good tendencies and sanctified his life. He has dwelt on the planes of fragrance and taste and is now ready to join the upward flow of energy in the fifth chakra.

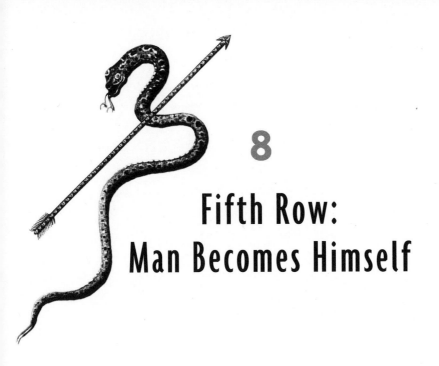

8

Fifth Row:
Man Becomes Himself

37
True awareness
(gyana; traditionally, *jnana)*

Knowledge of the right, and insight into the proper means of realizing the right in daily existence, are the two essential attributes of *gyana*. *Gyana* is an uplifting force, an arrow that takes the player to the eighth row and the plane of bliss, beyond the chakras. The player who understands his role in the game, and the nature of the course of action that will enable him to fulfill that role, lives in bliss.

The player realizes this wisdom only after the experience of clarity of consciousness. Only by suspending value judgments can the transmutation of energy that lifts him to the fifth chakra take place.

Gyana is not liberation. The player has yet to free himself from all those things that have clouded his mind. But he does know that the blocks can be removed, that Cosmic Consciousness is an attainable goal. Some Hindu philosophers see *gyana* as the direct path to moksha, Cosmic Consciousness. But in this game it leads to bliss. The player must still realize the plane of cosmic good and needs a throw of two to escape the cycle of rebirth. But there is nothing wrong. He can return to earth and play the game again.

Gyana then is awareness, not realization. *Gyana* is the understanding of the laws of existence and the awareness of a means to synchronize with them. The fourth chakra has already established balance; consciousness has been clarified. A true penetration into the world of concepts becomes possible. The player ceases to be attached to forms of expression and becomes drawn to the essence, the process of insight. Old relationships take on entirely new perspectives when viewed through the clear light of unobstructed consciousness. The cause of bondage is maya. The cause of liberation from maya to bliss is *gyana*.

As long as the player identifies himself as an individual, independent being he has karmas, and this is the cause of bondage. *Gyana* makes it clear that by reducing the scope and area of karma he can begin to establish himself in bliss. This is insight into the game itself.

In the first three chakras the player has been lost in the realms of delusion, fantasy, and power. Each course of action that inspired hope in him left the player in the end tired and painful. Finally, in the fourth chakra, he began to establish a sense of balance within himself. Then, with clarity of consciousness, he waded into the upward flow of energy that lifted him from the fourth chakra into the fifth. With balance, he sees his goal as attainable and adjusts his life in accordance with his insight into the process of fulfillment.

Gyana is a blank page. Whatever is written on its surface is only the illusion of *ahamkara*, ego.* Illusion is ever changing and thus is temporal. Only the page itself lasts, is atemporal. The page that remains after the writing has long since faded is *gyana*. This is the wisdom that makes the player understand the karmic writing on that blank page. To the degree the player desires, it is he who inscribes writing on his page. What

---

*The wisest course of action, then, would have been to leave this square blank. But there is an arrow in it. And, of course, the author feels the bliss of the experience, and he really cannot help expression, just as God could not when he said, "Let there be light."

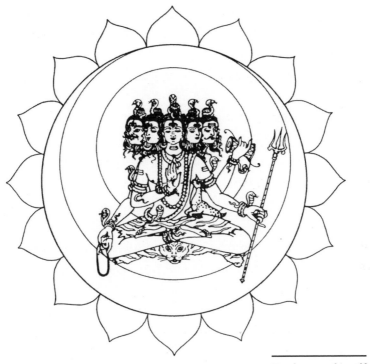

Man becomes himself

gyana dictates is that it be kept intact, handed over as it was given.

Gyana is rightly placed in the fifth chakra, because here is the source of those billions of blank pages that are the essence of the world's religious teachings. In the fifth chakra, communication with others becomes the main concern. The player seeks to convey the essence of his own insights into the game while simultaneously realizing the futility of the task.

38
Plane of life energy
(prana-loka)

Prana is *élan vital,* the life-force itself. In Sanskrit it is synonymous with life and is also the name of the lifebreath we take in with each inhalation. *Prana* is also the name of one of the five major airs in the body. As body air it is situated in the cavity of the mouth and enables food to pass through into the stomach. It resides normally in the area from the nostrils to the lungs, and its location near the heart preserves life from destruction.

Prana maintains the other elements of the body in balance and controls their function. With the help of *prana* we are able to move, think, see, and hear. From birth to death *prana* plays a crucial role in our lives: at birth it is the air that gives energy during delivery; at death it collects all vital energy from the body and flows out, leaving a lifeless corpse behind.

Prana is like a faithful servant, who fulfills all the demands of his master but in return does not demand any reward for his services. Like a true devotee, *prana* is devoted to the service of the self, consciousness, twenty-four hours a day. Yet *prana* is also temperamental. A slight change in the attitude of the master affects his speed and rhythm cycle. A good master, understanding the devotion of his servant, must try to help *prana* evolve. The methods to accomplish this are called *pranayama*, one of the most essential yogic disciplines.

In yoga, *prana* is of primary importance. With the practices of *pranayama* the yogi directs the flow of *prana* downward toward the pelvic plexus, where it mixes with *apana*, the air that resides in the lower intestines. When *prana* and *apana* flow together through *sushumna*, the central passage of the spinal column, to the top of the head, the experience of *samadhi* takes place—the goal of all yogic practice.

Prana is not to be confused with oxygen. The energy in the gross physical body feeds on oxygen. *Prana* maintains the existence of the physical body: *prana* is life. To understand *prana*, life and consciousness must be seen as distinct from each other. Life is a vehicle through which consciousness manifests, and *prana* is the energizing force of life. When life ceases, consciousness does not. This is evident from the many well-documented cases of rebirth.

39
Plane of elimination
(apana-loka)

While *prana* is the air that takes in energy from outside the system through the lungs and aids in conveying food energy to the stomach, *apana* serves the opposite function. *Apana* literally means downwards, and this is the air responsible for the elimination of energy from the body. It resides in the lower intestines; it expels the child from the womb and causes downward discharges of energy. *Apana* is the air responsible for urination, defecation, and ejaculation.

The importance of *apana* is poorly understood in the West. The presence of intestinal gases is acknowledged, but they are not even listed in a separate category or class. Scores of patent remedies are available for conditions brought on by disturbances of *apana,* but there is no understanding of their cause.

According to Indian medical science, *apana* is a great friend who aids in the cleansing of the system. The digestive process releases gases trapped in foods through the chemical interaction of the foods and digestive juices in the intestines. These gases are produced in greater quantity when the food is improperly digested, or when the circulation of juices has been disturbed (raw foods produce more gas, as do nuts and seeds). When, for whatever reason, the gases are disturbed, they start moving upward instead of down. This unbalances the chemical system of the organism. If the gases approach the heart they may produce high blood pressure, heart palpitations, and a heart attack. If they are driven still higher, disorders of the respiratory tract ensue. If the gases reach the head, schizophrenia results.

When *prana,* which is charged with positive ions, is made to function with *apana* and forced to enter through the central canal into the spinal column, a great fusion takes place between the positive ions of *prana* and the negative ions of *apana.* This generates a great amount of energy, which helps the ascent of the dormant energy at the base of the spine, called *kundalini*. (*Kundalini* is the immobile support of all the activities in the body. It is the energy that is present, in static or kinetic form, in all manifested phenomena. This is the energy used by the organism for its survival.)

By practice of the locks prescribed in yoga, *apana* is drawn upward. When it reaches the region of the navel it increases the gastric fire. Then *apana* combined with the fire of the third chakra pierces through the fourth chakra and mixes with *prana*. *Prana* is hot by nature. This causes a further increase in heat, and both airs rise upward, creating a vacuum. The scriptures say it is through this extreme heat, caused by fusion of *prana* with *apana*, that *kundalini* is awakened and enters into the central canal as a serpent enters its hole. This mixing of *prana* and *apana* rejuvenates the yogi, and he becomes a young man of sixteen, full of vitality, stamina, and power.

So on this square the player becomes aware of the importance of *apana* in his life and learns to keep the airs of his body harmonized through proper diet and other practices.

40
Plane of circulation
(vyana-loka)

Vyana takes *pranic* energy from the lungs and conveys it through all the bodily systems. It is the vital air responsible for blood flow, glandular secretions, upward and downward movements of the body, and the opening and closing of the eyelids. *Vyana* carries oxygen in the bloodstream into the capillaries throughout the system. Oxygen and *pranic* energy are absorbed by the tissues, and waste products are expelled into the blood. This deoxygenated blood is thrown out into the venous system by *vyana*. *Vyana* is also the force that carries this wasteladen blood back into the heart and lungs. *Vyana* produces sweating. We do not sweat only in certain special places but through each and every pore of the body. The only explanation for this is *vyana*. Sweat cannot move of itself. The air in the lungs cannot force it out, nor will the airs in the stomach, intestines, or anal region. What does, then? It is *vyana*—present throughout the body and crucial in balancing body chemistry through the processes of blood circulation, sweating, and coughing.

41
Human plane
(jana-loka)

Jana-loka is the fifth plane, the abode of *siddhas* (evolved beings who have powers by which they can do at will deeds that look like miracles to people who are on the lower planes) and saints, who are ever absorbed in contemplation on Hari. *Jana-loka* is also the region where inhabitants of *swarga-loka* and *maha-loka* seek refuge at the time of Great Dissolution of all existing phenomena, after which the universe is created anew. The element that predominates in this *loka* is air, and the bodies of the dwellers in *jana-loka* are composed of pure wisdom untouched by desire. This is the *loka* of divine wisdom, and those who dwell here are beings of divine wisdom.

The player who lands in the fifth chakra, the human plane, devotes his life to synchronizing with divine laws to sustain the upward flow of energy within himself. To stabilize himself in his experience he feels the need to communicate it to others. Thus the fifth chakra is the source of all great teachings. Its location in the throat near the voice box underscores the importance of communication to the player who vibrates here.

The player establishes himself here by a right understanding of the vital airs and by his passages through purgatory, clarity of consciousness, and *gyana*. His wisdom demands synchronization with planetary laws, and his understanding of the vital airs gives them the utmost significance. Imbalances in the airs are reflections of disharmony with planetary laws. Without the cooperation of these airs, synchronization is impossible.

His understanding of the divine presence within all existence, gained in his passage through the fourth chakra, demands he seek the Divinity within himself. Thus his attention turns to sounds, which take on a new significance for him. He is now able to hear sounds within himself that were inaudible before, because his attention had been aimed at the phenomenal world. Turning inward with his senses, he hears the sounds of his heart and the blood coursing through his system. These sounds open his nerves, and he becomes able to apprehend more.

While it has been said that all knowledge exists within, this becomes a reality only in the fifth chakra. The opening of the nerves produces sounds. These sounds in turn affect the psychic energy and result in changes in body chemistry. This produces a psychic state in which the player is opened to new dimensions of experience. The resultant understanding is known as knowledge.

In the fourth chakra the player has experience without understanding. The increase in energy caused by the elevation from the fourth chakra to the fifth elevates consciousness, and new perspectives come into view.

In the first chakra there are only four dimensions, called petals. In the second there are six. The transition from the second to the third chakra opens four new dimensions, and two more are added in the transition from the third to the fourth—a total of twelve. In the fifth chakra sixteen dimensions are functioning, giving a radically new perspective on the nature of the game. From this perspective all great religious teachings flow.

If the player who reaches the fifth chakra is part of a tradition, he becomes a new link in its development. Or he may leave and become an independent thinker, a seer, a prophet, or a saint.

This is the plane on which he gains a true perspective on the nature of humanity, and it is often gained directly from the third chakra by the arrow of selfless service.

42

Plane of fire
(Agni-*loka*)

Agni is a very clear manifestation of the eternal cyclic rebirth of the same divine essence. Fire is spirit, soul, and body at the same time. Our universe and what evolves within it, including man, are the products of the god Fire. In symbolic expressions he is shown with three faces, representing three fires—*pavak*, electrical fire; *pavamana,* fire produced by friction; and *suchi,* fire of the gods, also known in the Rig Veda as *vaishvanara,* the living magnetic fire that pervades all galaxies. The word *vaishvanara* is often used for the Self.

The player who lands in Agni-*loka* is ready to assume form. Agni is the fire-god; the fire is a gross manifestation of energy. In the body, this fire is life itself. It is love and security. It was man's security against the ravages of wild animals at the time when he lived in caves. But fire is but one manifestation of Agni. With air and water it is one of the three causes of the solidification of the earth and is thus the parent of forms. Fire is also the cause of light, which is a combination of colors. Thus fire is the cause of both color and form—the essence of the phenomenal world.

Fire is the gross manifestation of energy, its vehicle. The player who lands here understands that his body also is just a vehicle. For this reason, fire is regarded as the link between man and God. All religious rituals include the presence of Agni, the eternal witness. And because this fire-god is but an expression of man's innate nature, the player learns that self-deception is impossible. The witness is always there. The player who is about to take form does so with the knowledge that the role he assumes must conform to the dictates of planetary laws. Any deviation spells deception of the self, and a downward flow of energy inevitably follows self-deception.

According to Hindu mythology, Agni decided to explore the creation. He assumed an air-like form and traveled across the face of the universe on a lotus leaf. But after a time he grew weary and sought a place to rest. Soon he saw a nest on the face of the eternal waters. In the nest he spread his fire. The waters were the wives of Varuna, another manifestation of Agni. The fire-god's desire for these women flamed, and soon they were ready for union. His semen fell and became the earth. This is the fire he planted in the midst of the nest, and this planet is his offspring.

Modern science (i.e., Western science) now believes the earth to have begun as a ball of fire (Agni). Water cooled the surface of the planet, enabling life to arise. Even now, fire remains at the planet's core, as is demonstrated by the volcanoes that disgorge molten rock from the depths of the earth. Were this inner fire to die, life would vanish from the planet.

43

Birth of man
(manushya-janma)

Passage through the plane of Agni prepared the player for assuming form. *Manushya-janma* heralds the assumption of form. Conceived in the second chakra, nurtured and nourished in the third, filled with human emotions in the fourth, he now takes birth.

This birth is never registered in courthouses and hospitals. Rather it is seen in those who encounter him, who afterwards say, "We saw a Man." The player is now the son of nobody. Anyone could have been his father. He is the son of God only and belongs to no caste, creed, nation, or religion. He has no attachments and needs no identification papers or marks. He has found himself. Now he has taken birth. Now he can be felt. His presence is experienced strongly by those still taking birth. He has direct experience of truth, a face-to-face meeting with reality. He does not need to please anyone, because he has lost interest in cultivating a group of devotees and followers. He relates only with truth, and pleasing truth is his sole aim.

Man is a rational being. This faculty of reason helps him relate to the truth. One who lives out of harmony with the law of truth cannot be rightly called a man. He is some other creature in a human body, striving to take birth as a man.

44

Ignorance
(avidya)

The player who lands in *avidya* forgets the illusory nature of existence and becomes attached to certain emotional states and sense perceptions. This snake draws his energy down to the first chakra and the sensual plane. Loss of understanding of the nature of maya causes suspension of the rational faculty of the mind and leads to identification with certain states.

Vidya is knowledge; *a* means without. The absence of knowledge is ignorance. Knowledge is understanding one's role in the game from wherever one is at the moment. The real *avidya* is within the mind. No *avidya* exists outside the mental realm. Our perceptions of reality are but reflections of our own selves. But while nothing exists outside the mind, this does not mean that only the player and his mind exist. The world of name and form exists also, but it is perceived differently by every player's mind from the place where he is vibrating at the moment.

This same world is a place of enjoyment for some and a hell for others. Each mind receives the world in its own way and attaches importance to objects according to its own karmas. Real knowledge is to understand reality without assigning value judgments. Real knowledge is nonattachment to the objects of sense perception, which are always changing, temporary, and therefore not reality.

If the player only keeps track of his inner sound—the sound of his self, his being—he will not fall prey to his own mind. Mind is like a tiger dwelling in the forest of desires, surrounded by a reality full of prey.

Only by following his inner sound can the player escape the tiger and escape the fall back to the sensual plane. Otherwise he must start anew, finally to pass through the arrow of right knowledge.

Ignorance has rightly been placed in the fifth chakra, the fifth row of the game. Only where wisdom *(gyana)* is possible can ignorance exist. Ignorance accepts as the sole reality that which is only written on the page. So it is only when the player comes into the realm of knowledge and wisdom that ignorance can exist.

45
Right knowledge
(suvidya)

Whereas *gyana* is awareness of truth, right knowledge incorporates behavior (practice) with awareness, a combination that lifts the player to the eighth plane and the plane of cosmic good. He is now one square away from his goal. He attains the realization that he is a microcosm of the universe, an ocean in the form of a drop.

According to Hindu tradition there are fourteen *vidyas,* spokes on the wheel of truth. These fourteen are the dimensions of knowledge and contain all that is required for man to know and understand reality. These are the four vedas, six *shastras,* dharma, *nyaia* (logic), *mimansa* (critical understanding), and the Puranas. In an industrial society, however, knowledge has assumed a new guise. Now what is called knowledge has been reduced to the level of information, capable of being programmed into a computer. But human consciousness is more than a computer. Right knowledge requires experience.

Right knowledge adds to *gyana* a new dimension, the realization that past, present, and future are one; they are aspects of a single continuum. While wisdom can dictate one course of action, right knowledge can demand its opposite. Out of wisdom the disciples renounced

Christ. Out of right knowledge Christ allowed his own death—knowing that subtle principles always outweigh the value of material forms.

Right knowledge is the food of consciousness and saves it from the snakes of irreligiosity, sorrow, jealousy, envy, ignorance, violence, egotism, *tamas,* and the inert negative intellect. Right knowledge strengthens the inner voice. *Suvidya* tames the tiger of the mind and converts the forest of desires into a garden of interpersonal evolution.

Vidya comes from the root *vid,* meaning to know. The most ancient form of knowing was the state of *samadhi,* in which the answer is obtained by undergoing a direct experience of reality. Thus all Hindu knowledge is known as *darhan,* meaning to see or to experience. Knowing is becoming one with the object to be known. This is *vidya,* right knowledge.

With right knowledge comes the end of the fifth chakra, the fifth row of the game. The minute the player attains a full realization of the oneness of himself and the cosmos, he becomes one with the ultimate reality and reaches the plane of Rudra (Shiva), cosmic good.

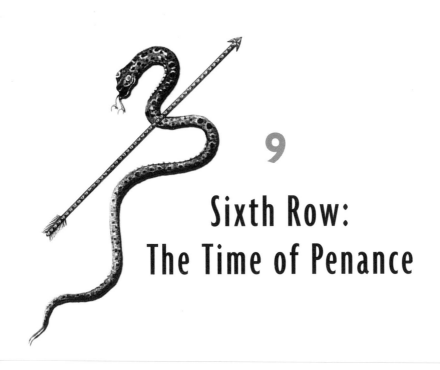

9

Sixth Row:
The Time of Penance

46
Conscience
(vivek)

Whatever exists in the phenomenal world is not reality. The objects of sense perception change with the passage of time, evolving, growing, and decaying. But these sense-objects give every appearance of being real. Man assigns value to the objective world and develops the desire for identification with these sense-objects. *Vivek*, conscience, is the power that saves him from falling back into the desire for attachment with the material. It is the player's own voice of inner wisdom that enables him to differentiate the subtle from the gross, to perceive noumenon in phenomenon.

Vivek could come no earlier in the game. The first square of the sixth chakra, conscience follows the passage through right knowledge. If the player lands on the arrow of right knowledge he is immediately boosted to the plane of cosmic good. Otherwise he has to take the help of his conscience in determining the course of play.

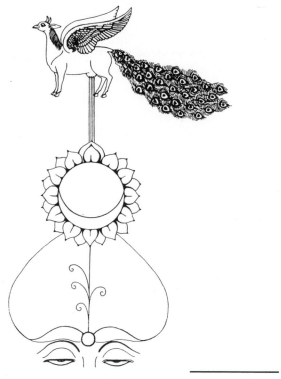

The time of penance

The basic elements of the phenomenal world are found up to the fifth chakra. These are the building blocks of gross manifestation. The presence of these elements influences the player's pattern of vibration as long as he operates from those chakras. But the sixth chakra is beyond the elements. Manifested maya now has little effect on consciousness.

When the player lands on the square of conscience he is immediately transported to happiness, a happiness that is possible only in the seventh chakra. In the seventh chakra the player is beyond all violence, which is cause for true happiness. But this is the sixth chakra, and here conscience is important. The sixth chakra has traditionally been called the third eye. Conscience is the third eye. Our two eyes see only that which exists—what was in the past, and what is in the present. But the third eye gives the power to discern future possibilities in the game, and that is one of the assets of the sixth chakra: insight into the future. This is no fantasy, but the direct perception of what will be.

Conscience is not something we grow in the course of a single, fleeting (by cosmic standards) lifetime. It contains the insights of the race in the form of the collective unconscious. The player has at his disposal a reservoir of experience within himself, which is now at the level of conscious awareness.

Conscience is the teacher that sits at the top of every player's head—the seventh chakra—guiding him throughout his life. The player can avoid social and political laws, but escape from the voice of conscience is ultimately impossible.

Before the player reaches the sixth chakra the notion of conscience makes little sense. But passage through the sixth chakra is determined by the fall of the karma die and the promptings of the inner voice of *vivek*.

47
Plane of neutrality
(Saraswati)

Psychic energy in the human organism flows through the central nerve canal of the spinal cord, *Saraswati*. According to yoga physiology, this energy flow begins in the first chakra and vibrates successively higher as the player advances from row to row. The ultimate goal of yoga is the raising of this energy to the seventh chakra, the crown of the head.

There are three basic types of energy in the human body: electrical, magnetic, and neutral. Electrical energy is sun energy and dominates the right-hand half of the body. Magnetic energy is moon energy and dominates the left. In normal states either electrical or magnetic energy (positive or negative, sun or moon) predominates. The neutral or psychic energy results when sun and moon are balanced in the body, when it begins to flow up the spinal column. Below the sixth chakra, control of this energy was not possible. Brief surges could be produced during meditation, but at seemingly random times and beyond conscious control. In the sixth chakra the negative and positive fade away; only neutrality remains.

When the player lands in *Saraswati* he comes into the realm of the goddess for whom it was named. He is surrounded by pure music and lives in a state of *vidya,* knowledge. The deity of learning and beauty graces him with the ability to stabilize himself beyond the influences of the electromagnetic field of existence. He has become a witness to the game.

Three nerves, which meet in the brain in the region of the third eye (between and slightly above the eyebrows), are responsible for the flow of the three types of energy. These are *pingala nadi, ida nadi,* and *sushumna nadi;* sun, moon and neutral; magnetic, electrical, and neutral. This juncture of nerves is called *prayag,* a name often given the third eye. *Sushumna* remains invisible, while *ida* and *pingala* can be seen as the two eyes. In Indian mythology, one of the most important holy sites is Prayag-Raj, the juncture of the country's three holiest rivers—the Ganges, the Yamuna, and the Saraswati. The Ganges and the Yamuna are *ida* and *pingala.* Both are visible, as are the two eyes. The river Saraswati is said to be invisible, flowing up to the *prayag* from the depths of the earth. This same symbolism is to be found in Greco-Roman mythology, in the form of the staff of Aesculapius, the divinity of healing. Two serpents twine around the central winged staff. The snakes are *ida* and *pingala,* the staff *sushumna.*

48
Solar plane
(Yamuna)

In the sixth chakra the player establishes a harmony between the male, solar principle and the female, lunar principle. This harmonious blending of the elements creates a witness-self, which is neither male nor female but a complete balance of both.

The solar plane is the plane of male energy. As long as a player is either masculine or feminine he cannot accept the opposite nature in himself, just as a player in a team on the playing field is unable to judge his own actions because his personal attachment to the game denies the possibility of right perception. But the one acting as the referee is beyond personal involvement. He is not committed to any team. He is the witness-self who is able to see the fouls committed by the player.

When the player vibrating in the lower chakras is tinted by the solar plane, his primary concern becomes destruction, power, identification of self—just as too much sunlight would burn the planet. To balance the sun, moon is needed. The player who lands here after passing through wisdom and right knowledge realizes this and learns to balance his own play of energies.

Below the sixth chakra solar and lunar energies entwine each other; but in the sixth chakra they meet and become one. This sense of oneness characterizes the plane of austerity.

To better understand the nature of solar and lunar energies and their function in the human organism, we have but to look at the example of the storage battery. Like a power cell, human beings have an anode and a cathode, positive and negative nodes. When both are placed in a solution capable of conducting a current, electricity is generated. The anode is positive and generally made of copper—which is red, a sun metal and aligned with the fire-sign Mars. For the cathode, zinc is used—a moon metal, bluish-white. The electrical charges gather around the anode, and through the anode we draw electricity. This electricity symbolizes the electrical (male) principle in the human organism.

In the human body the *pingala* nerve is synonymous with *Yamuna*, the solar plane. The solar energy is directly connected with the right nostril. When the right nostril is used, *pingala* dominates and there is a slight change in body chemistry, breath, and pulse. *Pingala* is the energy source for all creative actions and makes meditation impossible while the right nostril operates. In *pranayama* yoga techniques, the sun breath is often required. This simply means the aspirant should breathe through his right nostril.

Yamuna is one of the three holy rivers that meet at Prayag-Raj (now Allahabad) in the Uttar Pradesh province of northern India. Krishna was born near the banks of the Yamuna.

49

Lunar plane
(Ganges or *Ganga)*

The player who lands in *Ganga* finds himself at the source of magnetic female energy. He experiences the nerve *ida nadi*, located on the left side of his spinal column. *Ida nadi* is the source of the body's nourishment, attributable to its feminine (nutritive) nature. The female is magnetic, attractive; the male is electric, forceful.

The magnetic energy in man is closely related to psychic energy. The player who generates more psychic energy automatically develops a personal magnetism, which attracts to him those capable of being magnetized. Magnetism is actually a balance of polarity. Magnetic power is created by the interaction of the north and south poles of any substance capable of holding energy. The flow of energy from one pole to the other encounters no obstructions, and a magnetic field forms. In the same manner, an unobstructed flow of psychic energy becomes possible when meditation is practiced during those times when the left nostril, the moon nostril, is operating.

Through meditation the player lands on the lunar plane. Here he gains understanding of the female principle. He learns that a high tide in human emotions is reached on the night of the full moon, just as the ocean's tides reach their peak during the full moon. Both are the effects of the magnetism of the moon working on the planet.

Though the word *lunacy* was coined to note the relationship between lunar cycles and madness, the player who lands on the lunar plane of the sixth chakra need have no fears. At this level all energy is one, and female energy ceases to become destructive and becomes one of the most constructive squares of the game board. The left (lunar) nostril benefits not only meditation but music; dancing; enjoyment of poetry; removal of sorrow, pain, and depression; and restoration of consciousness. *Ida nadi* leads the player to the lunar plane, the plane of devotion and receptivity.

As a general rule, the left nostril should operate during the day and the right at night. The moon is needed during the day to compensate for the predominance of solar energy; and the sun nostril to compensate for moon predominance at night. This is the yoga of nostril breathing.

50
Plane of austerity
(tapa- or *tapar-loka)*

As knowledge was the main concern of the fifth chakra, hard work on the self—penance—characterizes the player who vibrates on the plane of austerity, the sixth chakra. *Tapa* means penance, mortification, burning and the practice of meditation on self-denial.

Tapa-loka is the sixth of the seven major *lokas*. This region does not perish at the night of Brahma. Air is the element that predominates in this *loka*, hence all the combinations interpenetrate each other without any difficulty. Although the elements finish with the fifth chakra within the human organism, in certain *lokas*, special regions situated in space, the elements still exist. Those who evolve by their hard work on themselves go to these *lokas*, depending upon the state of their consciousness. Those who dwell in this *loka* called *tapa-loka* are high ascetics and yogis—those who have gone on the path of no return and who are still engaged in high penances in order to be able to cross this level of consciousness and reach the next, the *satya-loka*, the plane of reality.

The developing witness-self recognizes the remaining karmas and sets about the arduous tasks necessary to burn them off. Hard penance is demanded. Karmas have become too heavy a burden to carry farther.

The player reaches *tapa-loka* either directly, through the practice of fourth-chakra *sudharma,* or gradually as he progresses through the fifth chakra, develops conscience, and masters his sun/moon energy system.

The experience of oneness with all reality strips the phenomenal, sensory world of its attractions. All the elements are now under the player's command. His insight into the nature of the space-time continuum enables him to see the beginning and end of creation. Living in this limited body, he becomes unlimited. The player knows he is immortal spirit in a temporal body. Death ceases to inspire terror. Here the player understands the meaning of "I am That" or "That I am," known in Sanskrit as *tattvamasi,* or *hamsa*. The player now becomes known as *paramhansa*.

Much is said in the West of the third eye. To understand this phenomenon, the player must undergo the rigors of the plane of austerity. He must do penance. He must get away from the identification with man or woman. His whole understanding of himself must change radically. He must recognize within himself the presence of the Divine. He must feel his own infinite nature. Here the sound *Om* becomes his mantra. This is the cosmic syllable that creates resonances throughout his system and helps raise his level of energy. Every hour of the day, every minute, he hears his inner sound. The sound grows more and more pervasive until it encompasses all the sounds in his environment, internal and external. Whoever is in his presence becomes calm and starts hearing the same high-frequency sounds generated by his own system.

Each player has a specific effect on other players, depending on the level at which he is vibrating at the time. The presence of the first-chakra man assumes either a terrifying or a pitiable aspect. He aggressively seeks physical survival or laments his inability to attain it. The second-chakra man, concerned with sensual indulgence, seeks to charm and soothe. His voice is seductive, unctuous. The player vibrating in the third chakra issues challenges. He asserts his ego wherever and whenever possible in the search for ever broader identifications and for confirmation of the aspects he has already assumed. The fourth-chakra player inspires those around him. He has found an emotional center and produces no threatening vibrations. The player in the fifth chakra holds up a mirror crafted of his own experience, in which other players can see themselves reflected. The presence of the sixth-chakra man reveals the Divine. The other players lose their identities and inhibitions and try to merge their consciousness with that of the one who has established himself in the plane of austerity.

51

Earth

(prithvi)

Earth is the great mother principle, the stage on which consciousness enacts its eternal play, Leela. Here the player understands earth as Mother Earth, not "the earth." The player discovers new patterns and harmonies, new ways of play, totally obscured before in the mists created by lower-chakra involvement.

Both Indian tradition and modern science agree that earth had its genesis as a ball of fire. What remained after the flames finished their job became earth. Earth is not only a planet but a living organism, the great mother principle who has given birth to all that exist on her breast. And as a mother carries milk, so does the earth provide nourishment, vital life-force, food, and energy.

Earth is the symbol of the sixth-chakra player. She is the product of great austerity. Her awesome birth by fire enabled her to give birth in turn to the live show of energy that is her mantle. She is the essence of tolerance and forbearance. Though her children blast her body and ignite her soul, she gives them in return diamonds, gold, and platinum. She follows the law of dharma selflessly and does not distinguish between high and low. Thus she is rightly placed in the sixth chakra. We see her body, the physical plane of the first chakra. What we cannot see is her spirit, her intelligence, her benevolence, her significance. This is the understanding that comes to the sixth-chakra player. He sees in her game the continual interplay of sun, moon, and neutral energies that mirrors the process always going on within his own microcosmic self.

Seeing inner reality reflected in the great mother, the player attains insight into Leela and becomes the Player. He must still pass through the plane of violence to gain an understanding of how to be truly fluid. But once these tests have been passed he may get a direct link with Cosmic Consciousness by landing in spiritual devotion.

Thus earth has nurtured her child-player to the point where he now has the ability to create his own game, to move higher or lower according to his karmas. Sometimes in the course of the game players rise up several levels as they experience the attributes of mercy, wisdom, and right knowledge. These arrows lift them to the highest plane. But since they really do not belong there, they are not assured of attaining Cosmic Consciousness. They have to make the trip anyway, and the game provides them with the snake of *tamoguna* to bring them back to earth, to make the effort anew. Each time the player goes higher and fails to attain the plane of Cosmic Consciousness, he must return home, to his Mother Earth—the cosmic playground.

And the more the player experiences earth, the deeper he appreciates the delicate balances that maintain life on her surface. To first-chakra man she is but a coffer to pillage and loot as he chooses, without regard to consequences. Sixth-chakra man recognizes the peril of this attitude as he sees the planet he loves facing imminent danger and suffering possibly irremediable damage.

52
Plane of violence
(himsa-loka)

The player who attains the sixth chakra realizes the unity of all existence. Human bodies are but transient forms. The real essence of all players exists beyond the realm of name and form. The player knows that death is just a change in the life scenario. Hence arises the danger that the player will resort to violent means, knowing full well his actions ultimately harm no other players.

But the world is the stage of Leela and karma. Each player has the opportunity of reaching Cosmic Consciousness within his present life. The law of karma dictates that all players must be allowed to enact their dramas to the end, to finish the play. Sixth-chakra acts of violence are not excepted from the omnipresent karmic principle. This makes the plane of violence a snake that draws the player down to fourth-chakra purgatory, where he must atone for his acts.

It has been individuals vibrating here who throughout history have launched the crusades, *jihads,* and other "holy" wars. The perpetrators of these vast pageants of human suffering and death always see themselves as great reformers of consciousness. Better the other player be killed than suffer his soul to live in ignorance, runs the rationale of the sixth-chakra zealot. After all, nobody *really* dies. . . .

Real violence is not possible before the sixth chakra. Acts of violence can be performed by players in lower chakras, but these are seen by the players as self-defense, as reactions to an external threat. In the sixth chakra players realize that no threat comes from outside. First-chakra violence arises over money and belongings. Second-chakra violence concerns sex and pleasure. The thirst for power creates violence in the third chakra. Fourth-chakra man kills to dispose of karma, to even old scores. Agnosticism is the fuel of fifth-chakra violence. In the sixth chakra establishment of a creed, cult, or religion inevitably provides the motivation for excessive force. Those responsible for man's unholy wars have been high ascetics, who have performed hard penances in order to gain powers. But if the karmas are bad, asceticism can lend itself to a sort of dangerous solipsism. The player believes he has *all* the truth—that he is, in fact, God or his agent. Those who fail to agree are wrong; therefore any means is justifiable to convert them. Better they die with understanding than live in ignorance.

In the lower chakras freedom of action is not present. In the sixth chakra the player becomes his own master and gains great powers through austerity and penance. Power in *himsa-loka* becomes violence. The player is violent with his own self before he can perform an act of violence on another. It requires perfect self-confidence to be violent. This self-confidence does not come before the sixth chakra. What had been reaction in the lower chakras is now nothing less than a sort of spiritual anarchy.

The player's lack of fluidity and spiritual devotion draw him down to even harder penances in purgatory, where he must truly repent from the heart to be able to go on with the game and seek the path of spiritual devotion.

53
Liquid plane
(jala-loka)

Water is cold by nature and absorbs heat, producing a sensation of coolness. The heat of the sixth chakra, austerity, makes the player violent. He has to pass through the pure waters of this, the liquid plane, to quench the burning energy of violence and convert it to the warm steadiness of spiritual devotion.

Water, one of the five elements, is the binding material of existence. Man's body weight consists primarily of water. In arid regions where water is either deep beneath the earth or nonexistent, the earth becomes brittle and fragmented, and we call it sand. Sand does not retain water. Water flows through quickly because the individual grains have no capacity to absorb moisture. The earth becomes barren, almost devoid of life. Water is therefore also responsible for fertility, germination, and growth. Growth itself is a process of heat, of fire. Heat provides color and form, and water adds stability. Water binds the form together and is the energy on which fire feeds. Thus fire "eats" water and provides the earth's vital energy, which is manifested as the life-forms of the planet's surface.

Water has no shape; it assumes its form according to the shape of the vessel. This is also the main attribute of the sixth-chakra player—the ability to become that which confronts the self. The real game starts when the player loses his identity as a player. Before the sixth chakra and the ability to become formless, the player has been caught up by money, sex, power, karma, and the search for knowledge. The game starts in the sixth chakra, when knowledge is obtained and the illusion of the form of identification of playerhood dissolves.

54
Spiritual devotion
(bhakti-loka)

Bhakti, or spiritual devotion, is based on the doctrine "Love is God, and God is love." A *bhakta*-devotee is in love with his Deity. The Deity is the beloved, and the devotee is the lover. The *bhakta* or lover experiences separation and longs to meet or even just glimpse his beloved. Nothing else attracts him; nothing else holds his attention; all else is meaningless. Food, sleep, sex, attachments, responsibilities—all are no longer important. He is dominated by his sense of separation and cries in ecstasy to have a glimpse of the Lord. When the *bhakta* is blessed by divine grace he feels an undivided union, and nondual consciousness prevails. He and his Lord then are one, and a Divine experience assures the devotee of grace that comes from the Divine.

Bhakti is the most direct method, the shortest way to experience the Divine. All yoga and knowledge, *gyana,* rests on the foundation stone of true faith, true devotion, true *bhakti.* There is nothing higher than love, and *bhakti* is the religion of love. Love is indeed God. To kindle the candle of love with the spark of knowledge, and to do the yoga of love, is *bhakti.*

In the final stage of the opening of the sixth chakra, when the player has become liquid and pure, he understands the real value of the game.

He understands reality both as it exists and as it appears. He knows the necessity of the plane of austerity, and of *gyana,* right knowledge, and *sudharma,* selfless service. He sees too that anger, conceit, nullity, sorrow, and ignorance are all meaningful aspects of experience. He is beyond all valuations. Everything has equal meaning and validity. He knows that as long as he remains in the body his karma die will lead him on his journey, stage by stage, square by square. He knows he will fall victim to serpents along the way, just as he knows he will find arrows as well.

All around himself the player sees the same game enacted by others, all passing through the same states at different rhythms and at varying intensities. He has attained stability in himself by mastering his will. For further development he now needs an emotional center for his life. To lose his identifications he can do nothing other than identify with the Divinity, in one form or all. One form becomes every form at this moment, the moment the player lands in *bhakti-loka.* In whatever form he finds the Divine, all other forms are magically present. The form literally becomes the Deity, which in turn becomes the devotee, an ecstatic *bhakta.* Earlier the player did not accept Leela—play—as his basic nature and remained caught in sixth-chakra vibrations until his energy accelerated too rapidly and became violent. But acceptance of Leela gives him devotion to the game itself.

He experiences the squares as a play of divine energy, and he feels oneness with each of them. They are all manifestations of his Lord. True *bhakti,* therefore, comes in the sixth chakra. Knower and known, subject and object, deity and devotee—all become One. In the sixth chakra the player understands this, and thus the many become a whole.

In the fourth chakra there is duality. Unity comes after knowledge is gained, in the fifth chakra. Without spiritual devotion the player begins to think in terms of an ocean. Spiritual devotion is the arrow that takes the drop to the ocean, after the drop has first realized the presence of the ocean within itself.

This is the only direct path to Cosmic Consciousness. The essence of Cosmic Consciousness could not be realized by sheer *gyana* or right knowledge. It is spiritual devotion that converts Cosmic Consciousness into a friend and gives a face-to-face realization of the Divine to the player. Knowledge and wisdom only provide an awareness of the cosmic principle. Devotion lets the player see the Absolute manifested in all experience. The Divine presence is everywhere, in everything.

Gyana makes a wise man out of the player, while *bhakti* makes him a divine child, ever in the warm lap of his mother and under the benevolent protection of his father. A wise man has to travel a long distance to see God. The *bhakta* is continually surrounded by the Deity in his myriad names and forms, in the sum total of life experience.

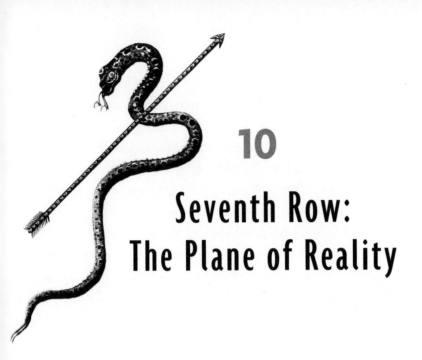

10

Seventh Row:
The Plane of Reality

55
Egotism
(ahamkara)

Aham means "I" or "I am." *Kara* (from *akar*) means form. When the I assumes a form it becomes *ahamkara*. When the center of activities in the player's individual self becomes his "I," then his *ahamkara* gets trapped in the maya of *me* and *mine*. When *ahamkara*—which is actually the highest aspect of reality—fails to identify with the whole and becomes a lonely part, then *ahamkara* becomes egotism.

When all the attentions of the player are directed solely toward attaining the object of his desire, the player becomes self-centered. Means are no longer important. The only good means are those, fair or foul, that hasten him to his goal. As long as he has humility and consideration, respect, and love for others, the means he adopts will have to make sense to him. He knows his own desires are not so important that they justify causing pain to another. But when desire overcomes the player's psyche, and he can no longer identify with humility, love, patience, respect, and consideration, he becomes an agnostic. He loses all sight of values in the here-and-now, by involvement in the karmas of establishing his identity in the game.

Melding with Cosmic Consciousness looks like a death to the ego. Old patterns, notions, and ideas must fall away if the player is to attain liberation. But *ahamkara* does not want to die. The ego wants to hold on to old identifications. This resistance increases the closer the player comes to attaining Cosmic Consciousness.

Hindu seers believe that sound is the source of all creation. Sound is the subtlest gross form in which energy existed before the creation. There are fifty-two forms in which sound energy exists in manifested form *(akar)*, and when the human organism evolved, these sounds localized themselves at the nerve endings of the psychic energy centers. The beginning sound is the simplest sound, *aa*. The last sound is *ha*. So all existence is from *aa* to *ha*. And the sense of identification that joins the *aa* to *ha* is *ahamkara*, the sense of being an individual self.

Yogis recognize consciousness in the human organism as having four primary aspects or categories: *manas*, mind; *buddhi*, intellect; *chitta*, being; and ego, *ahamkara*. All that is received as sensory perception is mind. The understanding of sense perceptions—their categorization and evaluation—is *buddhi*. The enjoyment and feeling of the sense-perceptions is registered upon *chitta*. He who thinks he is enjoying or receiving those sense perceptions as one person is the ego, *ahamkara*. When this ego becomes "the only one," every other thing becomes a means for the player to fulfill himself. Thus when *ahamkara* is not joined to Cosmic Consciousness it becomes egotism.

Ego is a direct effect of the feeling-self, *chitta*. In order to play the game, this feeling-self identifies with an object that moves from square to square, sometimes raised higher by arrows and at other times dropped precipitously by snakes. When the player totally identifies with the object, becoming elated with the arrow's rise and depressed with the serpent's bite, he is a victim of egotism. He is too attached to the object of play and has forgotten his own divine nature.

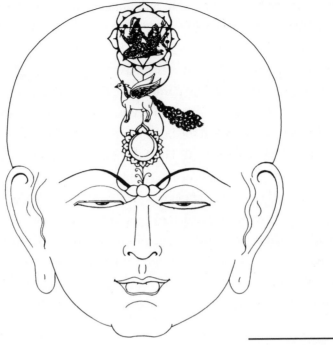

The plane of reality

This *ahamkara* does not exist before the fifth chakra, while the player is still in the process of taking birth. The fifth chakra is the plane of the birth of man, where *ahamkara* appears on the stage. The ego passes through ignorance and right knowledge and learns to hear the voice of his conscience as he enters the sixth chakra. But it is in the seventh chakra that the player really establishes his identity and begins to stabilize himself around an internal center. The player has found that he does not exist as a separate reality, that he is a manifestation of energy and must at some stage in his development merge with his source. It is here that the ego faces the danger of death and can turn into egotism.

The seventh chakra is the highest plane in the microcosm of the player. Here he reaches the peak and attains all that he has striven for. There are only two possibilities when one has attained a summit: merging upward in pure vibration and becoming formless, or falling. And the higher the player rises the farther there is to fall. If *ahamkara* fights the flow of *sud-harma*, anger is the inevitable result. This draws his energy down to the first chakra, where he must begin again his climb to the top.

Ego becomes egotism when the player is too self-centered.

In Hindu mythology the Puranas are filled with descriptions of this egotism, which was always reached after great penance and austerity. After the aspirant attained the boon of power, and became an egotist, he proclaimed himself to be God. This false identification drew him down to first-chakra anger, greed, delusion, vanity, and avarice. The whole planet became disturbed. Earth appeared as a cow before Vishnu and asked him to relieve her of the burden of egotism. At this point as described in the epics, Vishnu, the great protector of life, assumed a form by taking birth. In Leela, the God then sets out to slay the dragon of egotism in the player, an egotism contrary to the principle of preservation. *Ahamkara* is the food of Vishnu. Cosmic Consciousness is his dwelling place.

56
Plane of primal vibrations
(Omkar)

Om is the one sound present throughout the universe, manifest and unmanifest. It is the subtlest form in which energy exists. *Omkar* is the plane of the vibrations that produce this cosmic sound by remaining true to their dharma. The player who lands here discovers *Om* as the true sound of all being.

In the beginning there was sound, the Word. And the Word was with God and was God. This same sound can be realized by the player who abandons the trap of desires, which is mind, and meditates while creating sound with his body.

Om is the basis of all knowledge, all poetry, all the fine arts. Centering on *Om* opens to the player all the vast resources within himself, which were blocked out before by lower-chakra maya.

This same sound is also a great device for relieving tension. It is a sound used by every player consciously or unconsciously. For *Om* is the sound of humming. Everybody hums. Poets and composers, especially, make use of this sound to inspire creativity.

Om is at once Creator, Preserver, and Destroyer—the three aspects of Divinity. If the player finds himself associated with a disturbing element in his environment and wants to align himself with the harmonic rhythms of the planet, all he need do is start humming. The process makes him introverted, turning inward to unearth the vast treasures buried in the depths of consciousness, *chitta.*

If poets and composers vibrate in the lower chakras, their humming brings forth works that relate to that level of vibration. If they vibrate higher, their works relate to that higher plane. The Hindus believe that all the Vedas came out of *Om.* And it is clear that the Vedas were written by saints and seers who were also poets and composers already vibrating on high planes, for their work is the highest form of poetry, touched with the spark of the Divine.

The player who lands in *Omkar* has realized the need for creating calm in his life, for simplifying his existence. Worldly distractions have kept him away from *Om* and the cosmic wisdom it unearths. With the simplification of his existence, each action performed is performed consciously. The player ceases to be a slave of habit. As his being becomes more finely attuned to reality, he literally hums.

The humming process is *Om*-ing. This same sound appears in discussion when one affirms one is paying attention to the speaker. One makes a humming sound—Hmm or Ah. In the form of a sigh, *Om* relieves both pain and tension, and changes the body chemistry by driving out bad chemicals.

Humming vibrates the whole system, but most especially the top of the head—the seventh chakra. In the sixth chakra *Om* was the sound for meditation, for bringing the player into contact with reality. Here in the seventh chakra, *Om* is realized—a fact of existence.

The Vedic claim that *Om* enables the player to discover knowledge never present in his embodied life experience was confirmed in a study at the University of Saskatchewan. A group of 200 students chanted *Om* while trying to discover the answer to a question that none in the group knew. At the end of less than an hour of chanting, one in ten had uncovered the answer from the storehouse of cosmic knowledge that *Om* unlocks.

57
Gaseous plane
(vayu-loka)

Vayu-loka (literally, "the plane of air") is located in the region of *satya-loka*, the plane of reality, in the seventh row of the game board. This *vayu* is not the same wind or air as found on the physical or earth plane. It is the essence of the physical element air.

Marut is the ruler of this plane. He is also synonymous with Indra, the lord of Heaven (Indra is one who has obtained supremacy over his sensual nature). *Vayu-loka* is a plane where the player becomes a current of energy along which the whole atmosphere moves, obtaining supremacy over mass and weight. Those who dwell in this region are enlightened souls with a light body who have not yet reached the *satya-loka*, the plane of reality.

The player who lands in *vayu-loka* has made his passage through *Omkar* and achieved, through his karmas, higher vibrational patterns. *Maruts* are friends and brothers of Indra, controlling the atmosphere of the physical plane. They bring rain and fill the earth with the vital life-force. They become *pranic* energy on the physical plane and the life-breath of breathing souls. Air is synonymous with movement, inside and outside the body. All movements of fluids inside living organisms are due to air. Air is essential to life, and each and every cell has a vacuole (an air space). Air is thus present everywhere. The dweller in *vayu-loka*, being the life-force, life-breath, has the same quality as was found in the sixth

chakra: his presence can be felt anywhere, or in several places simultaneously. He can now dissolve the essence of his being, the ego, assume a
gaseous form, and float in the gaseous plane.

In the sixth chakra came the liquid plane, but liquid still has a form.
Gas, however, has no definite form at all. Liquid contains both mass and
weight; gas does not. The player is no longer burdened but he has gained
true freedom of action. He becomes weightless and formless.

58
Plane of radiation
(teja-loka)

Teja means light, and *teja-loka* is the plane of light. In the Upanishads,
self or consciousness is said to have four states:

1. The waking state, called *jagrat,* in which the self is known as
   vaishvanara.
2. The dream state, called *swapna,* in which consciousness is known as
   taijas or *tejas*—full of light, or made of light.
3. The state of deep sleep, called *sushupti,* in which it is known as
   pragya.
4. The altered state of consciousness called *turiya:* the unconscious/
   conscious state in which it is known as Brahman, Cosmic
   Consciousness.

Teja is the light that was created in the beginning. The world that we
experience in the waking state is the phenomenal world that comes in
the stage of creation before this. The phenomenal world is in the *teja*—in
the light from which it materializes. It appears to be similar to the world
of the dream state, but it is not. That state is completely made of light.
The images we see in photographs look exactly like the real person, but
they are different patterns of light, which vary to create an illusion of

reality. *Taijas* is related to the astral body *sukshma*, which is composed of light and in which the player dwells when he dreams.

To radiate is to emit light. *Omkar* is sound. After sound comes air, *vayu-loka*. And after air comes fire, *teja*, the subtle element responsible for all the forms of manifestation. Fire cannot exist without air, just as the player cannot land in *teja-loka* without first passing through the plane of air.

Every substance has a combustion point, a temperature at which it bursts into flame in the presence of oxygen. Heat is the excitation of molecules. The faster the molecules move, the greater the heat. Fire comes when this movement is too fast to be contained by the material. As the player rises higher and higher his own level of vibration increases. In the seventh chakra he reaches the essence of vibration. Then, his vibrations fully raised, he passes through air and bursts into radiant flame, giving light to all those around him.

When the player lands in *teja-loka* his light can be felt throughout the world. Though there are billions of stars in the sky, only a few are brilliant enough to be visible, and there is but one sun in each solar system. It is here that the player becomes light, illuminated. He becomes a sun, gathering around himself the astral bodies necessary to form a complete solar system.

The plane of radiation is not directly attainable by any arrow. The player must reach it slowly and gradually, unless he attains illumination through the practice of spiritual devotion.

59
Plane of reality
(satya-loka)

Satya-loka is the last plane of the seven main *lokas* seated in the spine of the game board. In *satya-loka*, *akash tattva* predominates: the player here attains the *Shabd*-Brahman world and is on the verge of liberation from the cycle of births and rebirths. He has reached the highest plane, beyond which lies the *vaikuntha,* the abode of Cosmic Consciousness. This *loka* does not perish at the night of Brahma, the Creator. *Shabda* is the word, the *aum,* which is itself Brahman (Absolute Reality, Cosmic Consciousness). *Shabd* Brahman is the plane of primal vibrations—*Omkar.* After passing through the plane of primal vibrations the player is able to establish himself in reality.

Satya is truth, reality, God. Here the player reaches his highest chakra and becomes reality, realized. Before this level the game is all a process of evolving toward this nature, his own true reality. The player who reaches here attains harmony, a balance with the forces of the cosmos. There are no obstructions to the flow of his energy.

It is here that the player becomes *satchitananda* (*sat* = truth; *chit* = being; *ananda* = bliss). He realizes that bliss is the truth of being. He stays in the state of *samadhi* as a drop rests in the ocean. He dwells in an ocean of bliss. His presence becomes divine, and he confers grace on other players.

Even here the player is not liberated. There are three snakes in the seventh row of the game. The first is egotism. The second is negative intellect. The third is *tamas.* By reaching the plane of reality the player has escaped one of these snakes, but two are left to contest his quest for liberation. If doubt or laziness remains, the snakes will pull him down.

But if the player stays in positive intellect, and his karma die leads him successfully past the snake of *tamas,* there remain happiness and the planes of the eighth row—and Cosmic Consciousness. He is aware of the dangers he faces, and he knows he must still perform right karmas to attain his goal. This is his realization on the plane of Reality. He realizes that not simply by vibrating in the seventh chakra will he attain Cosmic Consciousness. There are more karmas, more tests. There are no more arrows ahead of him, no more sudden upward movements of energy. He has to make his way according to his karmas.

60
Positive intellect
(subuddhi)

Subuddhi is right understanding, which comes only after reaching the plane of reality. After the player reaches *satya-loka* he attains perfect nondual consciousness and perceives the Divine in all phenomena. Nondual consciousness is real *subuddhi.*

As long as the player is in the body, intellect plays its part. It discriminates, distinguishes, and evaluates. In the seventh chakra these value judgments no longer relate to the outside world but turn inward to discern the player's own inner reality. Each judgment produces a change in body chemistry. These states are known as feelings.

When the player reaches Cosmic Consciousness his symbol, the ring (which is his body), loses importance. But until the sixty-eighth square is reached, the four faculties of consciousness—*buddhi, manas, chitta,* and *ahamkara*—keep working. *Ahamkara* in its negative phase becomes egotism. *Buddhi* also assumes positive and negative forms. *Chitta* remains in constant action and interaction with the three *gunas.*

Before reaching the plane of reality, *buddhi* does not become a self-existing phenomenon, and this is true for *ahamkara* as well. After the experience of *samadhi* in the seventh chakra, and the realization that comes from direct experience of the noumenon, *buddhi* starts analyzing and categorizing the experience. Here the direction can be either positive or negative.

The positive way of vibrating, *subuddhi,* is achieved by following the path of dharma, the source of the arrow that ends here. Positive intellect joined to the flow of the player's dharma are two of the most potent tools in the game to aid the player in his quest for liberation.

61
Negative intellect
(durbuddhi)

If the player does not follow the law of dharma, doubting the cosmic nature of existence and the divine presence in his every experience, he is caught by the snake of negative intellect and brought down to nullity.

He can neither relate to the lower planes nor call on dharma for help. He has to pass through all the second-chakra planes of vibration unless the arrows of mercy or charity intervene. Unless he gets the aid of the arrows he must atone for his negativity and find dharma again, or else chart an entirely new course of action.

Buddhi is at once a great trap and a great tool for liberation. As *subuddhi* it is a tool in the service of liberation. So *durbuddhi* is a downward spiraling vortex, which sucks the psychic energy back into the plane of the imagination.

Durbuddhi represents the negative valuations in the player that cause him to shut out possibilities. In order to reach his goal, the player must be able to accept whatever the world presents to him. If he denies any aspect, if he doubts the presence of God in any single object, he denies God. For the Divine is reality. All is the manifestation of the One. *Durbuddhi* is negation, negation of the Divine. This is why the player who comes here dwells in nullity. All his energies drained in his denial of God, he finds himself in futility. Until he can accept what he has denied, until he finds dharma again, he has no hope of liberation.

But nullity is a transient state. Cosmic Consciousness is the only absolute. And if the player reaches the seventh chakra again, his forced banishment to nullity can provide the insight necessary to maintain positive intellect and avoid the jaws of this serpent.

62
Happiness
(sukh)

A balance in body chemistry and psychic phenomena: that is happiness. *Sukh*, happiness, is a state the player attains through *vivek*, conscience, or by chanting *Om*, achieving *samadhi* and maintaining a positive intellect.

Sukh comes to the player when his conscience tells him that he is very near his goal, giving him the certainty that he is nearing liberation. The feeling he experiences is ineffable, beyond the power of words to describe. He feels the happiness of the river merging for the last time with the ocean after a thousand-mile journey, a feeling of merging with his source.

If in his state of happiness the player does not neglect his karmas and become lazy and inactive, there is a real chance of attaining Cosmic Consciousness within his lifetime. But if he is overwhelmed with the experience of happiness and fails to act, sensing his mission complete, the snake of *tamas* lurks just beside him, to swallow him and drain his energies back to the first chakra.

The game tells us he still needs a six to reach his goal, just as he needed six to take birth. But if he becomes lazy, if he feels there is nothing left for him to do, there lurk *tamas* and illusion.

True happiness is for the player who maintains his balance as he nears his goal. The game is important in its totality. His stable intellect enables him to discern patterns of flow, the current of dharma. He accepts whatever life presents to him. There is nothing he rejects. Even if he reaches the eighth plane and must come back again to earth, he feels the happiness that comes with knowing there is a goal that can be reached.

63
Darkness
(tamas)

In Sanskrit *tamas* means dark, relating to darkness. Darkness is an absence of light. Light is knowledge; dark is ignorance; ignorance is mind. And *tamas* has a second literal meaning in Sanskrit: it means snake. *Tamas* is a dark snake, the longest snake in the game, one that inexorably draws the player back into illusion and out of the illumination of the plane of reality.

In the seventh chakra, *tamas* is the ignorance that comes from attaching importance to sense perceptions. This ignorance comes after one realizes happiness and thinks that it is the end of the performance of karmas. But the player cannot stop all karmas. From happiness, the highest karma is a six, the lowest a one. Action cannot stop entirely.

Tamas is complete surrender to illusion. The player has lost sight of the never-ending nature of play. He has forgotten that until liberation is attained the game is not over. Inaction is an attempt to avoid the law of karma. Karma is dharma in action. The player who lands in *tamas* has forgotten that play does not stop in the seventh row and that by attaining *samadhi* he has not attained liberation. When movement slows in the upward direction, it must still be expressed—and the only direction from the highest chakra is down. The longest snake in the game awaits the player who neglects his karmas.

Three factors are at work in any event. The first is dharma, the essence of action. The second is karma, the action itself. The third is inaction, inertia, resistance. Because of the nature of the game, inaction triggers a downward flow of energy. Karmas are unavoidable. Attempting to avoid them is a karma itself, an action. Attempting to avoid karma is a karma that draws the player back to the second space of the game, illusion.

Tamas is synonymous with the state of deep sleep. When the sensory organs are completely withdrawn and awareness dissolves in sleep, the player is no better than a corpse, even though he is still breathing. In meditation, when all activities of the mind completely stop and the sense perceptions are drawn inward, it becomes easy for the player to slide ever so gently from the *sattvic* actionless state into the hypnogogic state, ending in deep sleep. For this reason *tamas* falls in the seventh row of the game.

It is here that *tamas* becomes a snake. At other spaces where he has vibrated, *tamas* has been necessary for the player. But here, in the plane of meditation (a form of inaction), *tamas* is a snake that changes the entire course of energy flow, drawing the player back to illusion. An attribute of *tamoguna, tamas* is the manifestation of the *guna* in the microcosm. When the same force is discussed as an attribute of *prakriti,* the phenomenal plane, it is known as *tamoguna.*

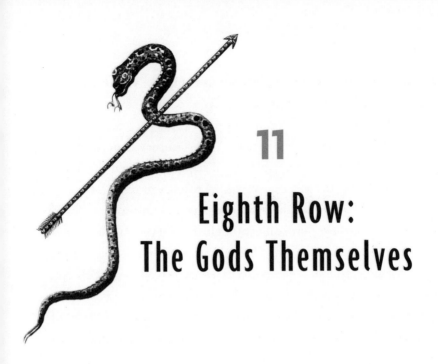

11
Eighth Row: The Gods Themselves

64
Phenomenal plane
(prakriti-loka)

Sri Krishna in the *Bhagavad Gita* defines *prakriti* as twofold: both manifested and divine. Manifested *prakriti* is the phenomenal world, composed of earth, air, water, fire, and *akash,* plus mind *(manas),* intellect *(buddhi),* and ego *(ahamkara).* This *prakriti* is eightfold and gross. The Divine *prakriti* is Maya Shakti. Krishna says to Arjuna, after mentioning the eightfold manifested *prakriti,* "Know my other *prakriti,* the higher, the life of all existence by which the universe is upheld." This is the imperishable *prakriti,* the will of the Supreme, everlasting and ever passing. This *prakriti* is beyond the seven *lokas,* beyond *akash.* The element predominant here is *mahat,* which is the source of all other elements: mind, intellect, and ego. *Maha* is "great," and stands for *tattva* (element), so *mahat* is *maha tattva*—the great element—from which the eight lesser elements emerge.

So therefore, gross, phenomenal existence comes from the divine *prakriti.* After the process of manifestation is complete, with the evolution of the individual self or man, a counter evolution starts—the self wants to reach back to the source. In this process the player starts from the physical plane (which he has reached in his journey from subtle to gross) and through karma and spiritual disciplines crosses the seven *lokas.* When he is able to overcome *tamas* he reaches *prakriti-loka.*

Up to the seventh level of the game the player confronts manifestations of *prakriti.* But after crossing through these seven planes he has gained experience and perspective. He is able to see what lies behind the world of sense-objects, and that is *prakriti.* Every percept has a concept. Concept without percept is empty; percept without concept is blind. Now the player draws near the concept, equipped with the percepts of his experience. Now he understands the fountainhead of phenomenal existence.

In Sanskrit *prakriti* means the original form of a thing, origin or source, material cause, the matter out of which anything is formed, a pattern, a woman, a mother. *Prakriti* is energy in its primordial form. It is energized consciousness, conscious energy in undifferentiated vibration. From this state develops the phase of consolidation of energy, of differentiation, of manifestation. Out of this state consolidated energy manifests itself in three primary dimensions:

1. The material content (which is also inertia, latent potential) that forms the body of the phenomenon.
2. Action and interaction in the process of evolution.
3. The purpose inherent within the phenomenon: the noumenon.

When the player lands in *prakriti-loka* after passing through the plane of reality, he is able to apprehend the three *gunas* and the five elements in their most essential form.

65
Plane of inner space
(uranta-loka)

After crossing the seventh row of the game and realizing the existence of *prakriti,* the player begins to merge into the source of phenomena, the great unenergized consciousness. At the moment of mergence all duality ceases. The player receives the pure experience of his own vast dimensions, the infinite space that lies within the Self.

Ur means the feeling self. *Ant* means end. *Uranta-loka* is the place where the feeling self ends, where all sense of separation ends. The player experiences the unfathomable depths within his own self. He finds the evolution and dissolution of all creation within the space of a single breath. He sees that all barriers are illusory. He has understood the nature of *prakriti* and realized the oneness that lies behind all manifestation. Now he is merging with that oneness.

Here there are no feelings. The witness-self has become fully realized. There is no good or bad, no vice or virtue. The player is a clear lens, allowing the passage of all light without restriction.

A description of *uranta-loka* can be found in the Puranas or Samhitas, works penned by seers and saints who experienced this space. They vividly described the cosmic knowledge that flowed through them. They became lenses of the lamp of pure knowledge, holding on to nothing, understanding everything.

66
Plane of bliss
(ananda-loka)

Consciousness is truth, being, and bliss—*satchitananda. Ananda* is the highest truth, the essence of being.

In the process of manifestation the Self is slowly covered by five

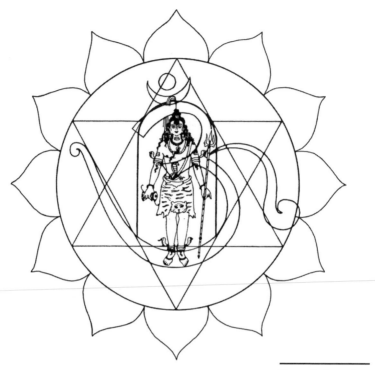

The gods themselves

sheaths. The first and most subtle sheath is *anandmayee kosh*, the sheath of pure being, pure feelings of pure consciousness. This is the sheath of bliss *(ananda)*. At the center is Cosmic Consciousness. During the period of manifestation this acts as the individual consciousness.

The second is the level of ego and intellect. This sheath is called *vigyanmayee kosh*. *Vigyan* is a combination of *vi* and *gyan*. *Vi* means beyond, *gyana* knowledge, *mayee* engrossed, and *kosh* sheath. This sheath, which deals with the knowledge of the beyond, is ego (which perceives itself as a separate reality) and the intellect (the evaluator).

The third is the sheath of the mind, the *manomayee kosh* (*manas* = mind). Mind works with the help of five sensory organs: the ear, the skin, the eye, the tongue, and the nose. From here comes all perception of the phenomenal world, the world of desires.

The fourth is *pranmayee kosh,* the sheath of *prana,* the vital life-force, the energy that operates through the five work organs and systems inside the body, including the blood vascular system, the respiratory system, and the nervous system, through which karmas are performed.

The fifth and most gross sheath is the *annamayee kosha. Anna* means the grain or food from which muscles, skin, teeth, blood cells, and semen are composed—the phenomenal person.

In the evolution of the inner self this process is reversed. The player goes through the *annamayee kosh* to the *pranmayee,* and crossing the four sheaths establishes himself finally in the sheath of bliss, the *anandmayee kosh. Ananda* is the chief characteristic of consciousness. It differs from pleasure, happiness, joy, and delight. These others can be explained, observed, and evaluated. They are relative states, which intellect can evaluate and categorize. *Buddhi* leads to *gyana,* the arrow that leads to the plane of bliss. *Ananda* is the primordial feeling of which all others are but manifestations. It underlies feeling and always exists at the heart of the player's being. But *ananda* can only be experienced directly, not observed in others. A deaf-mute cannot communicate the taste of a piece of candy in words. Only movements, gestures, and expressions can be employed. *Ananda* cannot be described or expressed; it can only be experienced.

In *uranta-loka* the feeling-self ended. All feelings became one when the world of sense-objects became one, since feelings are based on sensory perceptions. And *prakriti-loka* gave the player the knowledge that all sense-objects are but expressions of the one phenomenon.

Here but one feeling remains, the feeling of bliss. The experience of bliss is difficult until one achieves wisdom and becomes realized. The only alternative is devoting full attention to dharma while making the gradual journey up through the planes, avoiding all the snakes.

67
Plane of cosmic good
(Rudra-*loka*)

Rudra is one of the names of Shiva. Creation is the start of a threefold activity. It is followed by preservation of manifested forms and finally their disintegration or destruction. Each existing phenomenon is therefore going through the cycle of creation, preservation, and destruction. These three processes are ministered by the three powers of the one Creator, who is created by none and creates all. He creates from his will the Creator (Brahma), the Preserver (Vishnu), and the Destroyer (Shiva). The three are interrelated and interdependent. Creation is the divine will, and so are preservation and destruction. Without destroying the false identity—the concept of a separate reality, the individual ego—real union is not possible. Thus Shiva makes the individual consciousness one with Cosmic Consciousness.

Rudra is the lord of the south in the phenomenal world and is the furious form of Shiva. He was known as Rudra because he took birth from the cry of the Creator, Brahma. By his grace the mortals live, enjoy the divine game, create, destroy, or pay back karmas—the physical plane or phenomenal world being the land of karma.

Shiva also means good, good for all. He is cosmic good, alchemically changing magnetic into electrical energy and sending it back to the source. This evolution of individual consciousness is completed on the plane of Rudra. Here there is only one more step to union with Cosmic Consciousness. This is the *loka,* where the player's final purification takes place. This plane is beyond the manifested universe and is composed of the same element as *ananda-loka,* the plane of bliss.

Knowing, feeling, and doing are the three attributes of human consciousness. Knowing what? Truth. Feeling what? Beauty. And doing what? Good. For the player of the game, these three are the *summum bonum* of human existence. Good (being) is *chit,* truth is *sat,* beauty is *ananda: satchitananda.* By following the path of *satyam shivam sundarum*—truth, beauty, good—the player becomes *satchitananda*. These three aspects of consciousness are also known as *bindu, bija,* and *nada,* and they are worshipped as the three primary gods: Brahma, Vishnu, and Rudra.

Doing good requires knowledge of the right. Right knowledge can lead the player to the experience of cosmic good directly from the fifth chakra. The player who reaches here offers no resistance to the flow of dharma. He simply does his job, whatever the cosmic forces ask of him.

Rudra-*loka* is one of the three central squares of the uppermost row of the game. These spaces are the dwelling-places of the God-forces responsible for all creation, the forces with which the aspirant tries to identify. The player who seeks to identify with knowledge of the right finds himself in the abode of Shiva. Here he realizes the right, cosmic good. The essence of cosmic good is truth, while its form is beauty.

68
Cosmic Consciousness
(Vaikuntha-loka)

Above and beyond all other *lokas,* in the region of the beyond, is *Vaikuntha*—the *loka* of Cosmic Consciousness, the *prana* of manifested reality. This *loka* is also composed of *mahat,* the "element" that is the source of elements and not an element by itself.

Before the player starts to play the game, he accepts the importance and significance of this, the plane of Being, which is always his goal. Whatever desires lure him away from his path, this is always his highest desire—to attain *moksha,* liberation.

Vaikuntha is the abode of Vishnu and the plane every Hindu hopes to realize after passing from the present form of existence. The dwelling-place of Vishnu is the plane of Cosmic Consciousness because

Vishnu is truth, the great protector of consciousness throughout its upward climb.

The karma die observes the vibrational level of the player at all times. The die determines where the player must be placed and what course of action is to be adopted. The player can follow *ashtanga* yoga, the eightfold yoga, and evolve path by path through the eight levels. Or he can follow dharma and become a *bhakta,* a spiritual devotee. All paths lead to the same place.

Whatever his course of action among the limitless possibilities, the player has now arrived at the seat of Vishnu. And Vishnu is the essence of all creation, Cosmic Consciousness itself, truth. It is directly above the plane of reality because the highest reality is truth.

The ring that symbolized the player goes back to the finger of the one who wore it: it has lost all meaning. The game stops. What happens now depends on the player. The nature of cosmic play is simple. It is to discover by what different combinations, with what new karmas, with which companions can the player reenter the game and strive anew to seek the state that is his real home. He can continue the game of hide-and-seek with himself, or he can remain beyond the game for ever. Or he can go back to earth to see if he can help others reach the goal, thus taking the role of the twice-born *boddhisattva.* The choice is his. No one else can choose.

69
Absolute plane
(Brahma-*loka*)

On one side of *Vaikuntha* is the *loka* of Rudra, and on the other side is the *loka* of Brahma, forming the triad of Brahma, Vishnu, and Shiva in the middle of the game board, in the topmost row. This plane is higher than manifestation: the seven major and other minor planes mentioned and not mentioned on the game board. The predominant element is again *mahat.* Those who have established themselves in the truth dwell here without fear of going through karmic roles again, while those who practice mercy also reach the plane of Brahma, the Creator, and dwell there fearlessly.

Brahma is the creator of phenomenal existence. He is the active principle of noumenon, the force that energizes consciousness into the countless patterns and forms. His abode is Brahma-*loka*. The player landing here merges with this Absolute, this subtle principle. Brahma is the cosmic organizer who decrees the laws of form.

Though situated immediately adjacent to Cosmic Consciousness in the eighth row of the game, Brahma cannot liberate the player. Play must go on. Brahma decrees the form of the game, but there is more to the game than form. Truth alone can liberate the player. The three *gunas* await the player, and the serpent *tamoguna* must eventually take the player back to earth, the mother. He goes back to the sixth chakra, but not without the insight into the principles of the game that he attained in Brahma-*loka*. This insight can help him to his goal, and on earth spiritual devotion waits one throw of the die away.

70
True nature
(satoguna)

Sat means truth. When liberated, truth is Cosmic Consciousness. But this same truth, linked to the karma die, becomes subject to the three *gunas*, the three primary aspects of consciousness (*guna* means attribute). Attributes are qualifications of the player who is still linked to the karmic die.

Truth is the essence of existence. And in anything that exists the three *gunas* operate. Truth cannot exist of itself; it would then merge into Cosmic Consciousness. But the game is not finished; the ring is still there. So it is through these three *gunas* that consciousness will manifest itself for the remainder of the game. The player must return to earth and its game, both of which are products of the *gunas*.

Sattva by itself will create a state of equilibrium. Activity is required, and material to be activated. *Satoguna* is synonymous with light, essence, true nature, and vibration at its highest frequencies. The undisturbed state of meditation that gives rise to *samadhi* comes about when *sattva* predominates.

All that exists contains *sattva, rajas,* and *tamas;* yet nothing is purely *sattvic, rajasic,* or *tamasic.* As long as there is form, the creation of Brahma, all three are present. Only the proportions vary from moment to moment.

In the waking state *rajas* is predominant, while *sattva* is in the background contributing understanding and knowledge and enabling the player to act out his role.

In the dream state *rajas* is again predominant, and the dreaming self gets education from *sattva.* We never see darkness in our dreams; their light comes from *sattva.* Dreams are a process of purification, and in the dreaming state one is not bound by the laws of the physical plane. The player dwells in his astral body—away from and outside his physical body, yet connected with it by *sattvic* links.

In the deep-sleep state *tamas* is predominant, while *sattva* and *rajas* go into the background.

In *turiya*—the state of unconscious consciousness or *samadhi,* trance—the player dwells in pure *sattva.* When one is able to transcend the *gunas,* one is a realized being known as *gunateet* (beyond *guna*). These *gunas* are the dynamic forces that bring about changes in primordial *prakriti* and help the process of manifestation, becoming active when the cycle of creation starts. They are not three different entities but are interconvertible. *Sattva* during the process of evolution becomes *tamas,* creating sound, touch, sight, taste, and smell frequencies. The converting agent is *rajas. Tamas* in the evolution of consciousness becomes *sattva* in the same way, with the help of *rajas. Sattva* by itself is inactive and without the help of *rajas* cannot change. *Sattva* predominates on earth from twilight to three hours after sunrise.

71
Activity
(rajoguna)

Rajoguna is the activity in consciousness, or consciousness in activity. After reaching the eighth plane and failing to attain Cosmic Consciousness, the player is drawn on by karma, activity. This activity is the cause of all suffering. It predisposes one who is acting, and he is liable to fall prey to ambition and grow fond of rewards. Any obstacle in the course of pursuing a reward, or a desire, causes pain, suffering, and sorrow. When *rajoguna* dominates, pain and agony can be the result.

In *samadhi* the player dissolves *rajoguna* into *satoguna* and becomes pure light, *sattva*. If *rajoguna* remains, the player cannot attain *samadhi,* and *tamas* drags him back to earth. Because karmas accumulate and generate frequencies of vibration, these patterns take on form and become subject to the game.

As a *guna, rajoguna* balances *sattva* and *tamas. Tamas* tries to dominate *sattva. Sattva* tries to dominate *tamas.* Both are extremes of energy in *guna* form. *Rajas* tries to keep *sattva* and *tamas* in balance and makes the world of pleasure and pain, name and form, possible. No *guna* can exist by itself.

Rajoguna is active from three hours after sunrise to the evening when the sun starts setting. During this period the planet earth becomes active, and all the *karmas* concerning the preservation of life are performed. *Rajas* makes the player perfectly extrovert—and when he ceases to be an extrovert, *rajoguna* becomes an internal dialogue. Without conversation of *rajas* into *sattva,* the achievement of higher states of consciousness is not possible. By employing *rajoguna* in *sattvic* jobs one can remain in *sattva* while active.

72

Inertia

(tamoguna)

After sunset *tamoguna* predominates until twilight and puts the whole world to sleep. As *gunas*, *satoguna*, *rajoguna*, and *tamoguna* remain in primordial *prakriti*. After creation starts, *mahat* comes into existence, in which *satoguna* predominates. From *mahat* comes *buddhi* (intellect); from *buddhi* comes *ahamkar* (ego), which becomes *sattvic ahamkar*, creating mind *(manas)*, and *rajasic ahamkar*, creating *indriyas* (the sensory organs and work-organs) and *tamasic ahamkar*, creating the *tanmatras*. *Tanmatra* denotes that which is pure, not mixed. The *tanmatras* are five: sound, touch, color, taste, and smell. They correspond to the five great elements *(maha bhutas): akash*, air, fire, water, and earth. Combined, they create the individual self, in which these *gunas* are active in all four states of consciousness. Acting in the manifested world, they are not the pure *gunas* of primordial *prakriti*, for they have also become manifested. At that level, *tamoguna* becomes the greatest snake of the game board, *tamas*, at the end of the seventh chakra. In the eighth row the *gunas* are near the source and consequently purer.

The last square of the board and the beginning of a new phase of cosmic play provides the form, the material for the player. It comes in the form of a snake that bites the player and brings him back to earth.

Tamoguna is differentiated conscious energy. It contains light, but because of ignorance and lack of initiation it cannot evolve by itself. It needs *rajas* before the *sattva* within it will come out, reaching down to earth and taking form with the help of karma. *Tamoguna* veils the truth, making a serpent appear as a rope and a rope as a serpent. Darkness is the essential attribute of *tamoguna*, and inactivity its nature. The player who lands here immediately leaves the plane of cosmic forces and returns to earth to discover a new path to truth.

What happens is known only to the player and to the One who is truth.

Further Reading

Adyar, Dr. R. *Sanatana-Dharma*. London, 1966.

Aranya, H. *The Yoga Philosophy of Patanjali*. Calcutta: University of Calcutta, 1977.

Aurobindo, Sri. *Essays on the Gita*. Pondicherry, India: Aurobindo Ashram, 1972.

Avalon, Arthur. *Tantra of the Great Liberation*. New York: Dover Publications, 1973.

Blavatsky, H. P. *Secret Doctrine*. Edited by E. Preston and Christmas Humphreys. London: Theosophical Publishing, 1966.

Johari, Harish. *Dhanwantari*. San Francisco: Rams Head, 1974.

Sinha, Purnendu Narain. *A Study of the Bhagavata Purana*. Benares, 1901.

Woodroffe, Sir John, trans. *The Serpent Power*. Madras, India: Ganesh, 1964.

Woodroffe, Sir John. *Shakti and Shakta*. Madras, India: Ganesh, 1963.

Books of Related Interest

Numerology
With Tantra, Ayurveda, and Astrology
by Harish Johari

Chakras
Energy Centers of Transformation
by Harish Johari

Tools for Tantra
by Harish Johari

The Yoga of Truth
Jnana: The Ancient Path of Silent Knowledge
by Peter Marchand

The Yoga of the Nine Emotions
The Tantric Practice of Rasa Sadhana
by Peter Marchand
Based on the teachings of Harish Johari

The Yoga-Sūtra of Patañjali
A New Translation and Commentary
by Georg Feuerstein, Ph.D.

Shiva
The Wild God of Power and Ecstasy
by Wolf-Dieter Storl, Ph.D.

Kundalini
The Arousal of the Inner Energy
by Ajit Mookerjee

Inner Traditions • Bear & Company
P.O. Box 388
Rochester, VT 05767
1-800-246-8648
www.InnerTraditions.com

Or contact your local bookseller